Hot, NOT BOTHERED

99 Daily Flips for Slimmer, Trimmer, Fitter Faster

So You Can Master Your Metabolism Before, During, and (long) After Menopause

Debra Atkinson
Host of Flipping 50 TV and the Flipping 50 podcast

Voice for Fitness, LLC

226 Deer Trail Cir

Boulder CO 80302

E-mail: support@flippingfifty.com

Limits of Liability and Disclaimer of Warranty

The author and publisher shall not be liable for your misuse of this material. This book is for strictly informational and educational purposes.

ISBN-13: 978-1978089617
ISBN-10: 1978089619

TABLE OF CONTENTS

DISCLAIMER

The information presented in this book is not intended as medical advice or meant as a substitute for medical advice. Not all exercise is appropriate for all individuals. For personal exercise recommendations or nutrition needs seek the advice of an exercise or nutrition professional and let your physician know you are starting or implementing changes to your exercise or nutrition program that may have interactions with any current medications.

GENERAL INFORMATION

Despite what you may have heard, there is no substantive proof that weight gain, fatigue, or belly fat are mandatory parts of menopause and the second half of life.

DEDICATION

This is for every woman who is approaching 50 or who has already turned the corner on 50 who is ready for a different message about the second half of her life.

(No matter what your age, that is YOU!)

Everyone looks at a pretty girl. No one can take their eyes off a confident woman who radiates joy and energy.

That, is available to you as soon as you believe that it is and you're willing to use your mind, your food, and your movement to get it.

FREE BONUS

Because exercise is such an important part of mastering your metabolism and it's ideal to show along with telling you how to exercise, I created a special set of videos, recordings, and support for you.

This book bonus includes:

- how-to videos
- workout videos
- audio recordings
- a downloadable Interval Training workout PDF

They'll help you exercise simply, safely, and sanely.

You can get everything at:

https://www.flippingfifty.com/hotnotbotheredbonus

HOW TO USE THIS BOOK

The 99 Hot Not Bothered (HNB) "flips" include hormone balancing daily habits, exercise, and nutrition, and mindset. I began writing HNB as if the flips would be pajamas to pajamas. I strayed from that and you'll find some flips in the order to add to your day and then others that you plan one day and can implement the next day or next workout.

You can pick up HNB and flip to the middle of the book or read it front to back. We've already got too many people telling us how to behave, dress, or cut our hair after 50, so I'll leave this up to you.

"Flips" are the Flipping 50 way of changing a habit that is sabotaging you, or adding one you're not doing yet, with one that makes you look (and feel) 100% you. They are about changing the message you send yourself. They are about raising your expectations. They aren't about diet deprivation, the scale, or extreme exercise, or superficial beauty or flat abs tips.

One hint I share with all Flipping 50 clients and students is that if you get your "first two" right the other 22 tend to go much better. So if you're overwhelmed, focus on the flips in the front of the book.

Establish a HNB routine in the morning and you'll set yourself up for all day success. You'll have more energy, a better mood, more productivity, and you won't have to rely on willpower. You'll be full, satisfied, and have feel-good hormones rushing through your veins.

If you read all 99 flips today chances are you'll never implement any. I highly recommend reading a few at a time. Consider implementing before you go on and read more. They may require you to think or act differently than you do right now. They may challenge everything you've been told or learned. When new science replaces old science it can take time for our thoughts and attachments to old habits to catch up.

If you find yourself thinking, I've tried that before, it's probably true! You might, however, have randomly experimented in a way that it's impossible to know if something worked for you or not. If you start a new flip, commit to it consistently for a few weeks.

My hope is you find HNB is education, motivation, and inspiration. Each daily flip takes two minutes or less to read. You'll find an invitation to go deeper and get support throughout the book. My goal is not that you read the book but that you take action and find solutions you can easily add to your current habits for better results! Often ONE habit flip will cause a cascade of other good habits.

These are daily flips I use. They are flips I teach in all the Flipping 50 programs to coach my private clients. They are not random bits of information, but proven, tested, and results-getting flips that are safe, sane, and simple. The research is in the back of the book. Client stories are included throughout.

The most common frustration I hear from would-be hot women is confusion over how to move and what to eat. We collectively underestimate the positive power of sleep and the negative influence of stress. With clear tips inside for how to move and eat, and why, you'll have steps to change your workout ... or your lunch, today!

My biggest intention with this collection of "flips" is that you have hope for a flipping amazing second half and realize you are not limited by your age, or by hormones, or menopause. Nor do you have to be limited by your mindset. You are full of wisdom and vitality right now. You can enhance it and radiate joy. By doing that you will have a bigger positive impact on the world. That's hot.

Disclaimer: If you happen to purchase anything Voice for Fitness, LLC ("Flipping 50", "Debra", "Debra Atkinson", or "I") recommend in this or any of our communications, its likely Voice for Fitness will receive some kind of affiliate compensation. Still, I only recommend stuff I truly believe in, use, and share with friends and family. If you ever have an issue with anything I recommend please let me know. I want to make sure I am always serving you at the highest level.

Part I

Mostly Morning Flips

1. Wake Naturally

Beat your alarm clock to the punch. Waking naturally is a signal that your body has received a full night's sleep. You may be thinking you wake naturally all the time but it's more like a natural disaster when it happens at 2 or 3 or even 4 depending on your normal wake up. If you're not sleeping well you likely would love to comply with getting a good night's sleep but can't! If this flip is nothing else, it's a wake up call (pun intended) that you need to make a conscious decision to work on it. It helps your hormone balance and acts like the glue to make the exercise and nutrition flips stick.

Sleep is called an athlete's steroid. It's the same for you.

Getting a good night sleep starts with going to bed when you're body tells you it's tired. Test your sleep needs with my sleep needs test so you know. Optimal hormone levels by day happen with the right nighttime sleep.

Little details matter. The time you start sleep, end sleep, and the way you choose food and exercise throughout the day support or sabotage your sleep.

Just how important is it? One of my private clients was stuck for years with weight gains, losses, and plateaus. She made changes in her eating and exercise that made her a poster child for hormone balance. It wasn't until she was finally able to increase her sleep she unlocked the key to a 75 lb. weight loss, in her sixties. Even if you like Jennifer have had insomnia for years, it's never too late.

If you want support being an overnight success, get Sleep Yourself Skinny.

http://bit.ly/2fIdzCv

2. Drink Lemon Water

Start your day with a large glass of water with either fresh squeezed lemon or apple cider vinegar before anything else. You may not realize that overnight your body gets dehydrated. Particularly if you avoid drinking water in the evening so you don't have to get up for a bathroom break. By adding the lemon you'll also improve your pH level, give your digestion a boost, and support your liver naturally. Here's why that's important:

When you create a more alkaline pH, as opposed to more acidic, you give yourself a better chance to thrive. Disease loves an acidic environment.

Women, notoriously under report digestive issues and just live with them. No one likes to talk about poop, apparently. Eliminating is important! You'll feel less bloated and remove toxins from your body. This is a good first step for you if you're constipated.

Your liver is central operations for detoxing your body naturally every day.

If you're constantly under stress (welcome to reality), this little flip can be especially helpful. When you create a happy internal environment the outside comes along for the ride. Squeeze half a fresh lemon or add 1-2 T. of apple cider vinegar into to a glass of pure filtered water.

5

3. Test Your Drinking Water

Drink from a pure filtered water source to avoid fluoride, which is damaging for thyroid health. It's not the only thing to pay attention to but it's a big one! Your use of water is constant. Your drinking water, and water you cook with, shower, bath, or brush your teeth with potentially exposes you to toxins. Once in your body toxins are stored in fat making it hard to lose fat.

During weight loss if you have a significant amount of weight to lose you'll be releasing those toxins into your blood stream. They can interfere with thyroid function. Poor thyroid function can disrupt that weight loss. So it's important to:

- Reduce your exposure to toxins (test your water to know)
- Recognize signs you may be dumping toxins
- Support quick removal from your body when toxins are released (boosting fiber helps)

Signs of dumping toxins include nausea or fatigue. This feels like withdrawal from sugar or caffeine if you've done that it so it can be hard to tell the exact cause. Slow and steady weight loss will reduce the risk of a rapid toxin dump. You have all the time you need.

Don't assume that your water is fine because it's always been fine. Uranium was found in my neighbor's tap water recently. Uranium at too high levels in the water can lead to kidney issues. It's not one of the most common heavy metal concerns, but it's not ideal in your drinking water none-the-less. Lead, mercury, and arsenic are usually on the heavy metal hit list.

If you're chugging water daily to improve your health (yes, please!), be sure it is clean and pure! The same goes for water you're sitting in for that relaxing bath: it's crossing your skin and being absorbed into your body. I've switched to filtered water to be safe not sorry and I've opted to send a sample to a lab for further information on my own water.

If you find your tap water isn't up to par, consider bottled water or invest in a filter. Beware of water from plastic water bottles. The plastic contributes to toxin exposure. Never leave a plastic bottle sitting in the heat and go back and drink from it. Plastic leaches into the water and into you.

For more information on 8 habits that help you get more energy without even getting breathless get my tip sheet here:

http://bit.ly/2g7RVIz

4. Shine Early

Get some sunshine within minutes of waking. Direct sunlight is best but if that's not available get as much light as possible. This will enhance your melatonin production in the evening. The pineal hormone melatonin supports sleep. Both men and women produce less with age. On top of hot flashes, night sweats, or a mind that's working overtime you may be one of up to 60% of women sleepless in menopause.

Exposure to sunlight in the morning is one of the best ways to naturally boost melatonin production at night so you get a good night's sleep. This flip doesn't have to take additional time. Reset your body clock by taking your morning coffee on the patio or in bright lights.

If your schedule requires waking at o-dark hundred, at the very least turn the lights fully on. If you notice big mood swings with the weather, you may be more sensitive to light/dark changes. Consider investing in a light box and use it daily.

Sleep is crucial to mood, memory, and weight loss that is fat not muscle. Get more tips for sleeping yourself skinny.

http://bit.ly/2fIdzCv

5. Clean Up Your Coffee

If you drink coffee, choose organic. Avoid flavored. Drinking more than one cup? Drink a glass of water between. Recently, coffee consumption, provided it's not laden with sugar and consumed all day in search of artificial energy, has shifted to a less negative position on health. Some studies even show it may prevent several chronic diseases. Coffee drinkers unite!

Moderate consumption – under 3 cups providing 300-400 mg/d of caffeine – shows little evidence of health risk and some benefits.

More than 4 cups a day will contribute to your risk of low bone density. It's not just the coffee consumption but what you're not drinking that might negatively impact your health. If sleep is an issue for you try cutting back to two cups a day.

Personal secret: caffeine has long been an ergogenic aid in exercise. If you're enjoying your java pre exercise it may boost endurance and fat burn during that run or lift session. It's more beneficial in longer sessions than in short HIIT sessions. So if you're doing a moderate steady state session followed by weight lifting or if you're headed out for a longer hike, it might be a good time to try it.

To use caffeine strategically for a workout boost, exercise about 60 minutes after consuming coffee. If you're sensitive to coffee and elevated blood pressure added caffeine might not be a good choice for you however.

Should we talk about the elephant in the room? Worried about the diuretic effect of coffee interrupting your workout? Once your body adapts, as long as you don't wait too long between drinking coffee and beginning exercise, you should be fine, or at least your norm will be true. You won't be any worse off.

6. Cream Better

Flip to Medium Chai Triglyceride (MCT) oil or coconut milk (coconut cream is my favorite) and stevia. MCT oil is good for fat metabolism and doesn't get stored as fat. Bonus!

Why? Even if dairy doesn't seem to be a problem for you, it's tolerated less well by women in midlife and beyond. That can mean bloating and gas, signs that would motivate anyone to give it up, that you may not even be associating with dairy. It can mean weight loss intolerance. Even that little bit? Yes. Constant regular exposure to it is like having an IV drip coming in. Your gut can't heal when that's happening, so even small regular amounts, at least until you remove them for a period of time, can prevent you from feeling your best.

Add ghee, or clarified butter, to your coffee if the MCT doesn't appeal to you. It could change the way you think about coffee forever. More importantly it could change the way you think. Healthy fat coupled with the caffeine kick could make your morning more productive, and help you be less distracted with hunger pains.

7. Cup Down By 10am

Your goal is natural energy. Feeling like you need a caffeine fix may be a sign you need something else. Leaving coffee alone the rest of the day may improve your gut health and your sleep. Whether it's the ritual and the warmth, the caffeine buzz, or something else, waking up to a little coffee is fine for most. Depending on coffee to get you through the day is not.

Soda drinker? Get used to saying "I used to drink pop. Now, I feel so much better."

Sorry, there's never a good time for soda. While there is evidence that coffee can have positive health benefits there is zero health benefit and many health risks associated with soda consumption.

A trick that works for many of my clients weaning off soda is sparkling water with a few drops of stevia. Infuse your water with fruit or make a simple lemonade with fresh squeezed lemons and stevia.

Even if you opt for decaf coffee, limit yourself. Water is so much better for you. The biggest energy boost is going to come from real health not a cup.

8. Be Back Smart

Wait an hour after you rise to exercise. The wait protects the discs in your back. Any exercise including the stretching exercises you may have once been taught to do before you get out of bed can be more dangerous than you think.

If you're used to pulling your knees up to your chest before you rise, hold off on that. Bending, lifting, and twisting (BLT) movements especially in that first hour after waking can be devastating. Even in gentler exercises that are involved in yoga, Pilates, and vigorous walking you're at risk. Don't even think about core exercises during this time. It's not about the speed of the movement or the quality of your technique. It has nothing to do with whether you're fit or deconditioned.

Exercise stresses on the spine are about three times higher in that first hour than they are a few hours later.

After rising from bed, your discs are fully hydrated and have much higher stresses during flexion. It is more risky to train repeated bending earlier in the morning. Occupational studies have shown avoiding flexion motion in the morning reduced disabling workplace back pain.

It's not just movement though. There are two types of stress to the discs. Both movement and moment stresses the spine. That is both flexion (movement) that you would do in a crunch or downward dog for instance and simply the pressure (moment) of adding force as in doing a plank or pushing a shovel or vacuum. Both strain the layers of collagen in the spinal discs.

When loads on the spine are small, movement is healthy. (E.g. cat cow back) This is the type of exercise to begin your day with rather than extremely vigorous exercise.

If you feel a little stiff in the morning, a better way to relief if you're tempted to stretch before getting out of bed is to simply tighten and release muscles throughout your body. Think of making a fist and releasing. You can do the same with your feet and leg muscles and so on. You'll bring some blood flow to them without risk. Circle your feet and your hands and shrug your shoulders. Then carry on.

The shape of your discs and the thickness of your spine determine how much you're at risk for herniated discs. Do you know the shape of your discs and thickness of your spine? Few people do until it's too late. There's evidence that you have a limited number of forward flexion no matter what the status of these two variables. It's a matter of whether you move toward injury faster or slower with forward flexion and BLT combined movements.

If you've been an early morning exerciser, this flip is not good news. Maybe you've just found time to journal, or read, or start writing that book. Within an hour of being upright 90% of that extra disc fluid dissipates and exercise becomes much safer.

This would be so much easier to accept if you could feel the damage. No one has to tell you to avoid painful movement. The problem with disc damage is you won't feel the damage happening until it's too late. It's worth a shift in your schedule so you can keep exercising. If exercise helps you negate stress it's even more important that you make shift in your morning routine so you can continue to be active.

9. HIIT It Early

It may not matter what time of day a young man does interval training. For you, however, the earlier in the day you can do intervals the better. Here's your motivation for early intervals:

- Boost your fat burning potential
- Enhance rather than interfere with your ability to sleep
- Offset your body's newfound ability to store belly fat

You feel a significant amount of stress compared to men, or younger men or women. You may have excellent coping skills and maybe you're the exception to the rule. If you compare your mid-life self to your younger self, while hormones are up and down and all around, there's a good chance you're "feels like" rating of stressors is higher.

Cortisol is naturally elevated in the morning, at least if all is well. It begins to fall in the afternoon and by night it's low, so you can go to sleep.

You may not need me to tell you that sometimes that's a dream. Your circadian rhythm can get off. High intensity exercise early can help you reset this rhythm. Its one of the best ways to balance the bad boy stress hormone that can team up with insulin and increase fat storage.

Both high intensity intervals and or intense weight training done in the morning boost your energy, cognitive function, and fat burning all day, too. If you are fatigued first thing in the morning, waking up feeling like you've got a hangover without having had the fun, less is more. Even 10 minutes of high intensity exercise early in the day can boost your energy level all day.

There's another hidden bonus in morning exercise. Most women tell me that they are more active later in the day even if they've started with a small dose of exercise early. A body in motion stays in motion. Just taking a few extra steps, or adding dog walk after work increases your activity level in important ways. This kind of Non-Exercise Activity Time (N.E.A.T.) is more related to obesity and overweight risk reduction than your gym session.

Can you exercise later? Yes. Later is an ideal time to do lower level activities that reduce stress. If you have difficulty sleeping, vigorous evening exercise can make things worse. Rapid Eye Movement (REM) sleep is important in restoration. REM is decreased by 10% with evening exercise.

Yoga or a walk with a partner, pet, or your lovely self, for instance are good examples of late day exercise. Even weight training done later in the day if you must as long as you keep a watchful eye on your exercise and sleep quality connection. A session on your own or just you and a trainer instead of that extreme late day bootcamp are good late day flips.

Are you stuck with a schedule that means those early morning high intensity workouts are not going to happen? Make the most of your weekend. Then reassess your thoughts about how long it has to take.

For 14 months, I was limited to 20 minutes of intervals or weights. I had been a fitness instructor and endurance athlete for decades used to doing hours a day of exercise. After 14 months, I felt better, looked better and was the same weight (in fact, slightly lighter) and body composition I'd been when I was spending far more time exercising. If you have two weekend days and you can get up 20 minutes earlier one day during the week, you too can get more results in less time.

The interval training (IT) PDF inside your book bonuses outlines simple IT options you need to get and keep you slimmer, trimmer, and fitter faster.

https://www.flippingfifty.com/hotnotbotheredbonus

10. Go Pro

Make your first meal of the day a high protein breakfast. A breakfast that included 35 grams of protein voluntarily reduced subject's daily calorie intake by 400 kcals. Study participants weren't asked to make the change. They did so voluntarily not intentionally. They were simply sated (the no thank you, I'm comfortably full, factor) and the high protein breakfast influenced their entire day, not just morning.

Whether you're intermittent fasting and breakfast is later in the day or it's first thing, a high protein meal has the power to improve your choices at your next meal. Say bye-bye to cravings and take back your power over food. Add high fiber foods at the same meal and you have a winning combination for energy and won't be distracted by a growling stomach. The added bonus is a reduced insulin response to your meal. That means, less fat storage and greater fat burning.

I used to be a dash-out-the-door-girl with coffee and nothing. Not so coincidentally I also used to flirt with regular stomach issues and irritable bowel syndrome (IBS). When I started having a smoothie for breakfast 20 years ago, the gnawing feeling in my gut I was so used to disappeared. I had better morning runs, made better choices at lunch, and my afternoon energy soared. No more IBS.

Smoothies are not the only way to get your protein in. They may be the most convenient and delicious. Get 60 of my favorite smoothies and the formula I use for creating my own every morning.

http://bit.ly/2kiavC9

11. Time Food Right

Wait 60 minutes after intense workouts (either strength or cardio) to eat a high quality protein meal. There is a blunting effect that happens immediately after exercise that prevents muscle protein synthesis from occurring. After about an hour this blunting effect is lifted.

The best time to eat a high protein meal is 90 minutes after intense exercise. This may not be possible all the time. Do the best you can with the schedule you have. A little planning ahead goes a long ways to optimize the time and energy you put toward your exercise program. The results you get depend on the trilogy of exercise, recovery, and nutrition. During menopause when things beyond your control can go wrong, get control of the habits you can.

If you're habit stacking and you're a morning exerciser you may be thinking this is all fine and good if this is all you have to do all day. Are you wondering how you wait an hour to exercise after you rise, exercise, then wait another hour to eat and still go about your day? That's a perfect day. If you can't stack them all every day, focus on what you can do. With a short intense workout and a shake to go with you, it may be easier than you think. Here's a sample morning schedule:

- Rise at 5:30am
- Exercise 30 minutes at 6:30am
- High protein meal or smoothie between 8 and 9am

Flipping Point: remember that three of the most common mistakes women make around exercise is nutrition: eating too little, eating the wrong thing, or timing it wrong. Even "healthy" foods at the wrong time can sabotage your flip.

12. Aim Higher

Plan higher protein meals for you did for your younger self or do for younger family members as a rule. Older adults don't synthesize protein as well as younger adults. A higher amount of protein post-exercise now than when you were younger (40 grams) will help you keep the lean tissue you're working so hard to create and spare muscle losses that can occur with age or following exercise breakdown.

If you notice you've lost muscle tone or struggle to get muscle back after losses due to inactivity or illness, this is even more important to you. If you're not just flipping 50, but sizzling at 60 moving toward 70, it's more true for you, too.

Sounds like a lot, right? You don't have to do this all day but post exercise the difference in exercise success for older adults vs. younger adults was comparable if the older adults had increased protein following weight training sessions. Without the additional protein boost older adults exercise benefits were less than younger subjects experienced.

A smoothie with a high quality protein shake mix and a serving of nut butter can easily add up 30 grams of protein. Read your labels. Other protein boosts include hemp hearts and chia seeds. If you prefer, eat some smoked salmon or bacon.

You'll notice I don't recommend yogurt, dairy or soy milk. These are protein sources but 90% of Flipping 50 program participants find they lose weight, bloat, improve energy and feel better when they remove these. I don't know about you and neither do you until you test them. Beware that whey is a common protein shake ingredient and that may also contain casein. These two are dairy. So until you've tested I would avoid them all.

The right amount of protein at the right time will help prevent muscle loss that sabotages your goals. Get clear on your protein needs with the Protein Report recording in your book bonuses!

https://www.flippingfifty.com/hotnotbotheredbonus

13. Supplement smart.

Take a multivitamin delivered in at least two doses over the course of the day that is formulated for optimal absorption and low competition. Those little micronutrients apparently fight for a spot to land and there are only so many receptor sites.

Supplements also offset daily habits that deplete micronutrients and compliment your eating preferences by making up for nutrients you're not getting in food. Whether you're vegan, vegetarian, or go Paleo, or a blend, your individual habits leave you void or lacking some specific nutrients. It's not just a special diet that does this. None of us can eat as much as it would take (20,000 calories or more) to get all the nutrients we need on a daily basis.

Good habits like exercise also deplete our micronutrients. Prescription medications and over the counter drugs also deplete you of micronutrients. They do their job and then some.

A liquid vitamin, or one that's powdered and stirred into liquid could bump your ability to absorb all the goodness. You're a machine. You need all the parts working to have a healthy metabolism, good digestion and powerful immune system. Cravings, lack of sleep, and belly fat might be a result of missing micronutrients.

This is one I like. http://bit.ly/2jyla7n

14. Get Sugar Smart.

Avoid fructose, sucrose, sucralose and all other natural and artificial sugars in foods as a rule. Natural sugars like honey, cane sugar, and agave have the same effect on your body as white table sugar. Especially post exercise if you're trying to lose body fat or increase your lean muscle tissue, these ingredients will increase your storage of fat.

Sugar aliases like maltodextrin and dextrin (and dozens of others) as well as artificial sweeteners, which are hundreds to thousands of times sweeter than sugar and addictive are prevalent on ingredients labels you might never suspect. Those hundred calorie packs of nuts, and even protein powders you may be using to get lean contain them. Artificial sugars create the same insulin response in your body and make you more at risk for diabetes regardless of your body weight.

Even small amounts of sugar can sabotage you by continuing to nurture your taste for sugar. Start reading your labels and tossing those items that are backfiring your health goals. What you'll soon realize is that "sugar content" can be high even when there is no added sugar.

Stevia is the safest alternative to date. It comes in powders and liquid form. You may want to try a couple brands before you give it the thumbs up or down. Try to wean yourself from too much of the sweet taste. Your taste buds turn over in about 11 days. If you can leave it alone for just that long you won't long for it any more.

15. Hypnotize Yourself

Put yourself in a positive trance. You know that little voice of doubt inside your head? The more often you put positive messages in to count it, the better. You have two chances every day. Spend time in the last hour before bed and the first hour upon waking with positive thoughts, meditation or journaling, to set a positive mindset in action.

You're in a hypnotic state during these times and your creativity is highest. Start and stop your day with gratitude and expectations about what you want to manifest. It's a powerful habit. Your brain stores memories while you sleep so why not take advantage of influencing it.

You may hear more about toxins in your environment from electronics, skincare products or drinking water, but your thoughts can be toxic, too. Start purging them now. You may not realize until you start to write them down or you try to meditate for a few minutes just how often something negative comes into your mind.

There are some common denominators when I'm working with women. We tend to think we're flawed. Do you ask questions like, "What am I doing wrong?" In the heat of the moment (if you don't get it the first time), do you say, "I'm so dumb!" or "What an idiot?"

Negative self-talk related to exercise and diet usually sound like this:

- I have no discipline
- I'm just lazy
- I'm not very motivated

Sound familiar?

The words you choose really matter. Nowhere are they more important than when you're talking to yourself!

When it comes to a simple, affordable way to change your life and course of every day fast, this is it.

16. Break Up with Make Up

Your skin is the largest organ in your body. Choose your personal hygiene products carefully. If you've already explored this one, you're way ahead! Regularly sweep through your make up drawer, soaps, lotions, and hair products. If you travel frequently don't leave it to chance and use whatever the hotel might have available. If you shower at the gym a few times a week be sure your gym bag is packed with toxin free products too.

Body washes, lotions, shampoos, and toothpaste can contain toxic ingredients that act as hormone disrupters. Many of them are referred to as obesogens that can cause weight gain and impede weight loss. They cross your skin and are stored in body fat. If you use products that contain these chemicals daily you increase your toxic load. That makes it hard to lose the fat.

Start by reading your labels armed with a hit list of items you don't want anywhere near you. Know where to look for clean, chemical free products. Environmental Working Group's site www.ewg.org is a good start. Head to the resources list in the back of the book for more lists of good, bad, and ugly ingredients.

For your first flip, replace any product containing fragrance, toothpaste with fluoride, and shampoos or lotions with parabens for safer products. Choose safe and environmentally conscious brands designed for your skin now.

Fluctuating hormones can cause breakouts or dry, thinning skin. Does it feel like Monday it's wrinkles and Tuesday it's breakouts? If skin issues are causing you to rethink your routine this is one of my personal favorites.

http://bit.ly/2bZSD8F

17. Keep Your Promises

Set a daily appointment for regular exercise. The most important relationship you have is with your body. Some exercise requires recovery and some exercise is recovery. Exercise some days can consist of simply stretching while other days will be very vigorous.

Create a lifelong habit by setting aside a regular time dedicated to movement. Things will come up and change your schedule, but it's always easier to move something that's a normal part of your routine than to add it to your already jam-packed life. Exercise doesn't happen if it is left to a time when it's convenient. When you stop thinking of exercise as optional it becomes the norm and not the exception. Your best exercise partner is consistency.

If you don't believe you have time, you do. How much time do you think it takes?

If you don't know what to do, I've got you covered. Join me for a 5 Day Flip. I'll shoot you a simple checklist of the exercise priorities for getting hot, not bothered in less time. Then I'll send you five days of short videos so you don't have to make a single decision beyond lacing your shoes and clicking play.

Convince yourself that you can do it.

http://bit.ly/2kluW1l

18. Kill Cravings

If you're constantly reaching for a snack to satisfy a craving, start tracking your fiber. If you're weight loss has stalled though you seem to be doing everything right, start tracking your fiber.

Fiber and protein together kill cravings. Fiber is also essential for good digestive health and that helps remove toxic ingredients from your body. The daily fiber recommendation for women over 50 is 21 grams/day. Most Americans get an average of 15 grams of fiber a day. Remember that daily recommendations were created to prevent disease. To thrive your personal fiber best may be more. Increasing your fiber beyond the daily recommendation is suggested for anyone who wants to lose a significant amount of weight. Between 35 and 50 grams may be most supportive of weight loss and disease prevention.

Don't randomly start increasing your fiber. Once you've determined what you're current fiber intake is, then gradually increase by 5 grams/day from your current total. Maintain that for 5-7 days while also maintaining or increasing your water intake if you have room for improvement there. Your body will adapt to small incremental increases comfortably. Fiber from foods is best, because it contains a natural variety of fiber sources. If you do add fiber with a natural supplement seek a balance of soluble and insoluble fiber to avoid potential harsh effects of fiber due to a single source of fiber type.

Start with food. Eat fiber-rich foods at each meal. Nuts and seeds, leafy green vegetables, legumes, berries and avocados are loaded with fiber. If you're doing that and still not reaching a goal range, then consider a fiber supplement. Toss a scoop of fiber into your morning smoothie or add it to soups to boost your intake.

One of my favorite craving killers is a Mint Smoothie that tastes like your favorite Girl Scout cookie.

Chocolate Mint Smoothie

Chocolate Paleo Power or Plant Power Protein Shake

½ frozen banana (eliminate to cut down on sugar)
¼ avocado
handful of spinach
1 T raw cacao powder
1 tsp Mint Greens
1 tsp Fiber Boost
Small amounts of unsweetened almond, cashew, or coconut milk to thickness
Ice (especially if you're not adding frozen fruit)

Make it thin and drink it or thick and top with:

- Cacao nibs*
- Sliced almonds
- Raw

Flip: Add the cacao nibs directly to the smoothie after you blend for a mint chip smoothie experience.

It really is a thin mint treat.

http://bit.ly/2yKi8nr

19. Bust Your Rut

Variety is key. Eat a variety of nutrient-rich foods daily. Vary your intake day-to-day. It's so easy to get stuck in a rut and eat the same foods day-in day-out. Those foods you tend to have daily are the ones you are more likely to become sensitive to which can cause "leaky gut." That leads to gas, bloating, and constipation or diarrhea.

Beyond those unwelcome symptoms, however, the bigger concern is that you're not absorbing nutrients from healthy foods you're eating. You could be weight loss resistant if you're not getting all the nutrients a healthy body needs. Your body needs all cylinders firing to work properly.

Flipping 50 Fact: Even healthy foods can cause toxicity. Spinach, for example, is one of the most nutrient dense foods on the planet, but it's best to rotate it with other greens. Include kale, baby greens, and chard or romaine lettuce n your menu for diet diversity.

Your body does like routine. Diversity within routine is what you're striving for here. If you have fruit for breakfast, have strawberries one day and blueberries another. If you add greens to a smoothie or eat lots of salads, rotate with the options above. That helps you get more nutrients overall.

Get a diverse selection of micronutrients from vegetables in by eating different selections from each of three groups daily: leafy greens, the onions-mushrooms-cabbage group, and deeply colored vegetables.

If you snack, have a few options that work for you instead of going to the same thing every day. For instance, have nuts one day, boiled eggs or veggies with hummus the next, a cup of bone broth on another day.

Write it all down for three days. Then read it as if you were going to hand it in to me as your coach. You'll already see areas for improvement.

20. Stop the "Carbage"

Don't ditch carbs completely.

Include complex "low and slow" carbohydrates at every meal. Increase the number of carb servings at each meal throughout the day. Start with a lower carb breakfast and have the most carbs at dinner. Shocked? Here's how to make sense of that.

Cortisol levels ideally peak in the morning and fall throughout the day. When cortisol drops you can become more edgy. If calming carbohydrates increase as cortisol decreases you'll avoid that "hangry" feeling.

If you have a hard time getting adequate quality or quantity of sleep pay special attention to your carbs. Eating the largest portion of carbohydrates at your evening meal will calm you with some serotinin and help you get a better night's sleep. If you're in the habit of decreasing your carbohydrates at night to help prevent weight gain, and you're not sleeping well, this small change by itself may improve weight loss. More carbs for weight loss? Who knew?

All carbs are not the same, however. Choose low and slow. That is, low Glycemic Index (GI) and Glycemic Load (GL) foods that are released slowly. Quinoa, brown rice, legumes, and sweet potatoes are good examples.

Want more support? Check out the Flipping 50 28 Day Kickstart.

http://bit.ly/2xTVKv9

21. Flip On Fat Burning

Our public health attitude toward fat has changed significantly in the last 20 years. If you're still playing the no or low fat game, flip to moderate or full fat options. Science is discovering the benefits of eating fat for losing fat and maintaining optimal body weight.

What's the secret to fat burning? If you want to reduce mood swings caused by blood sugar issues, and want to become a fat burner as opposed to a sugar burner it requires a combined exercise and nutrition approach.

Once you've adapted to better quality carbs (Flip 20), begin to reduce your total carbohydrate intake and increase your fat intake, paying attention to your energy needs and how you feel. Too low a carbohydrate intake can have the same effect on your body as too high a carb intake. Find the sweet spot where your mood, focus, energy, and weight management feel easy and effortless. You'll feel best when you find your personal best carb intake.

Choose high quality fats. Chocolate cake doesn't count. Guacamole, salmon, and olive oil do. So do nut butter and hummus. Aim for about 5 servings of fat a day. As hard as it may be to release the old idea fat makes you fat, it couldn't be further from the truth.

The once vilified saturated fats are not as damaging alone as we thought. It's in combination with carbohydrates that easily turn to sugar that heart disease became a bigger risk. Eliminate excess processed empty carbohydrates and enjoy satisfying fats as a part of your diet again.

While you're in the increase fat, decrease carb phase, build a good aerobic base by exercising slightly longer than your norm at a lower level without eating carbs beforehand. If you constantly supply your body with carbs that's what it will choose to burn. There isn't a reason to dip into fat storage.

This shift of energy burn to fat from carbs will make you more metabolically efficient. You'll use fat for fuel, enjoy more stable energy, and if food is constantly on your mind, you'll get your life back!

22. Count On Protein

Flip 10 emphasized the power of a high quality high protein breakfast. It's not the only meal where you need to count on protein for flipping 50. Studies show between 20 and 30 grams of protein three meals a day is optimal for muscle protein synthesis (MPS). MPS is the amount the body can use at one time. It's not too much or too little. Track your per meal goal instead of a total at the end of the day or a total by body weight.

If you're thinking that you have less need for protein because you're not active, I have news. Even if you're sedentary you need adequate overall calories and adequate protein to avoid muscles losses with age. In fact, active women synthesize protein better than inactive women. That means the requirement for protein is slightly higher per meal for inactive than for active women.

If you're active you may be fine as long as you get 20 grams of protein per meal. If you're less active and or healing from an injury, you may require closer to 30 grams of protein per meal.

If you are highly active or you're having trouble gaining muscle in spite of exercise you may also want specific amounts of protein pre (24 grams) or post exercise (up to 40 grams) to prevent muscle breakdown that occurs due to exercise, aging, and without adequate nutrition.

Susan started following this advice the first week we began coaching. At our second meeting she was raving about how much more energy she had. The real intent of increasing protein to adequate levels is the long-term benefit of preventing muscle loss. Yet, if your levels are far below where they should be you too could find this little immediate gratification.

Listen to the Protein Report recording in your book bonuses for more details.

https://www.flippingfifty.com/hotnotbotheredbonus

23. Go Coconuts

Add medium chain triglyceride (MCT) fats to your diet. These fats are hard for your body to store and increase your body's ability to burn fat. That's a two-for-one I can wrap my head around!

They make food taste great! Coconut oil, coconut cream, and coconut milk are great ways to bring more MCT into your life. You can use coconut oil to add an Asian flavor to foods as you cook, substitute coconut milk for cream in soups instead of milk, or top your berries with coconut cream.

Most of my clients report feeling sated and more energetic during their exercise when they increase their consumption of fat. After losing 38 lbs. in four months, one of my clients said, "… and I did it without being a slave to the scale" or "letting food run my life."

You may recall the scare about coconut oil in the news recently. My friend and health expert Dr. Steven Masley answered questions raised recently by the American Heart Association (AHA) release. According to Steven, at this time the evidence is inconclusive about whether coconut oil causes heart disease. The problem seems to be when it's consumed with inappropriate carbohydrates. Nonetheless, Dr. Masley's advice is if you have an existing heart condition err on the conservative side and use other healthy fats, like avocado oil and olive oil.

If you are apparently healthy and enjoy the Asian flavor coconut oil offers you may have another source of resistance. it may feel strange. For so many years you may have shunned fat and associated it with gaining fat.

It was the best science of the time and new science has replaced it. Your thoughts and habits will catch up. It's a delicious and satisfying habit to catch onto. I start early by adding MCT to my coffee! Try it!

24. Handle Snack Attacks

Tune into your need or desire to snack. If you're hungry 1-2 hours after a meal, physiologically your body shouldn't need anything, so it's a sign. Check on the contents of that last meal. There should be protein, fat, and fiber in each meal. If you've had adequate amounts of each and you're still "hungry" not just craving something that's a sign you may have a blood sugar issue. It could also be that you're leptin resistant. Leptin is the hormone that tells your brain you're full after a meal and you're fine until the next one.

You want to get to the root cause of why but don't make yourself sick doing so. Start flipping snacks to those things that can help improve blood sugar naturally. Be proactive by including healthy snacks like avocado or turkey slices for instance to stabilize blood sugar and avoid a crash. If you do crash, though, you'll need some carbohydrate to help you feel better. As you improve your overall diet and decrease empty carbohydrates and high glycemic index foods (included fruit, especially dried fruit), the better you'll feel. Regular exercise, both cardio and strength training, is effective at helping stabilize blood sugar levels.

25. Hydrate Right

Find your personal best water intake. The old average of 8-8oz glasses of water a day is just a good starting point. Recommendations now focus more on your size. Take your weight in pounds and divide in two. That's the number of ounces you should drink. Some of us need less and some of us need more.

Environment or exercise can affect our own personal need on a day-to-day basis. The most obvious signs you're not getting enough water is thirst. To get an immediate read on your hydration, look at the color of your urine.

If your skin lacks a glow, you're constipated, lack energy or you're fatigued to the point you want to take a nap in the afternoon, it could be other things but the fastest most basic fix is to drink more water. .

To increase your water intake find your average daily intake by tracking for 3-4 days. Once you have an average, add a single cup more daily for an entire week. That is, if you've been drinking about 2 cups a day, for the next 7 days try to reach 3 cups a day. The following week, shoot for 4 cups a day and so on. Allow your body to gradually adapt and you won't have to run to the bathroom so often. Your body will put the water to use.

If you're worried about getting up in the middle of the night slow down a little on your water consumption. Spread it out evenly over the course of the day. As you slowly increase your intake every cell in your body will start using it and operating better. You'll be eliminating less frequently.

If you're not motivated to drink more water, here's a flipping 50 fact. A body under stress stops burning fat and stores fat easier. If you're dehydrated, your body is stressed. So, reverse engineering this principle, by staying hydrated you can enhance your body's metabolism and ability to burn fat.

Once caveat: drink your water between and not at meals. Consuming large amounts at meals interferes with the digestion and absorption of nutrients in the meal. Drink first thing in the morning, between meals, and have one last glass before bed to stay hydrated round the clock and enhance your body's ability to use food for your health.

Cheers!

26. Be That Girl

What did you eat today? Where were you? How much did you move today? How congruent are the foods you ate and the exercise you did with the results you want?

If you really want to master metabolism you want the best-for-you food. You can test and control that easiest at home. But it's not impossible to do when you travel or eat out either.

You want to plan to be active and stick to it with a plan B or even C that is your minimum standard. Even when it's not convenient. Is getting up at 4am convenient? No. Will it disrupt your roommate or your host if you're traveling? It might. Do you know that doing that when you're at a conference sitting for hours on end can make all the difference in how you feel when you land back home?

Be high maintenance for a change. Honor your needs.

On a recent client call I talked with Donna Thursday night. She had been at a conference all week. She was exhausted; "Spent." That was her word. She hadn't had enough water. She drank coffee to keep herself awake during boring sessions. She didn't exercise while away. The food wasn't what she would have chosen.

First and foremost, she needed a mindset flip.

No one is going to prevent you from carrying a water bottle. No one is going to hold you down and make you eat food you don't want. Put a water bottle in your suitcase and bring it. If there isn't water in the rooms, there are water fountains or a gift shop nearby. Find water. Bring an in-room breakfast option or snacks that will supplement a meal in case there's something you don't want to eat.

Had she gotten 10 minutes of movement in the morning in her hotel room, and started drinking water after morning coffee she would have felt much better (and been more alert).

Today it's pretty common upon registering for a conference that you'll be asked if you have any special dietary needs. Say yes. Ask for what you need to feel good.

I have friends and clients who travel almost every week and look and feel amazing. My best friend recently lost 50 lbs. He's 62 and has to eat every meal except breakfast out due to job responsibilities. Every one of these individuals has overcome a health or weight problem. They've come come up with different ways to manage eating well while traveling that include:

- Cook ahead and carry small food containers in insulated bags (airline approved)
- Stop at a grocery store before ever arriving at hotel for fresh food in room
- Travel with small cans of sardines and almost fresh avocados
- Find favorite whole and healthy restaurants in cities they're visiting and they have their food delivered
- Order using the menu as a suggestion. No sauce, marinade, or dressing has to come because it's listed!

You'll reduce your exposure to preservatives, food left out too long in restaurant buffets, and prepared with ingredients you're trying to avoid like gluten or grains, soy or dairy. Have you identified the foods that could be sabotaging you?

No matter where you are meal planning is the key. At home pick recipes full of good-for-you ingredients. Shop, prep and eat them.

"I don't have time to plan." Is that what you're thinking? You do! Buying, eating, and preparing food happens one way or another, planning doesn't take much more time. It will give you time back in the energy you have. It will end the last minute what's-for-dinner trauma.

I know what that's like, too. I was a single mom, running between two big time consuming jobs, and getting a kiddo to and from school and sports. Sure, I caved on occasion too. Never once did I feel better physically after eating out instead of cooking a better meal at home.

Step-by-step:

- Define foods that make you feel good.
- Find recipes that feature flavors you love made with your feel-good-foods.
- Make a shopping list.
- Set your shopping date.
- Set a prep date for yourself or people you'll share the meals with.

Once you establish a higher standard norm at home, you can keep it easier on the road.

Fast flip: Plan your meals today. Write down what you've had so far. Now plan the rest of your meals the best you can with the information and options you have right now. As soon as you take charge of this you take charge of your energy, sleep, skin, and belly fat!

"Eating healthy" is not the same for everyone. It's not even the same for you today as it was 10 or more years ago either. If you're looking for a diet or meal plan before you identify your personal needs, it's going to fail you. You either won't lose weight or you'll regain it and more when you're done. You've got to be a "lifer" that's committed to finding your own personal best. You need a blueprint not a one-size-fits-all diet, or exercise program.

Forever flip: If you don't know what to eat, and you want support learning how to find out so you can eat more and exercise less, jump right into the 28 Day Kickstart.

http://bit.ly/2xTVKv9

27. Know Beans About That

Beans are an excellent source of fiber and plant-based protein. They're often the brunt of jokes and blamed for gas, bloating, and worse. Here's the simple solution. Soak your beans and legumes before you eat them. So yes, that means buy them raw and cook them instead of buying canned. You won't be sorry: they taste so much better this way.

This is especially for my vegan readers, but it's for anyone trying to bump fiber and plant protein for better health. Soaked or sprouted beans and legumes foods (and grains) are easier to digest. The enzyme inhibitors in beans not soaked are often the cause of the bloat or gas you experience after eating them.

Internal effects of beans can be more than embarrassing. You may be sensitive to lectins, which can damage the intestinal wall. That means you may be eating a stellar diet but not absorbing much of the nutrients in the food you eat. Soaking or sprouting beans, legumes, and wheat can help.

How to: soak dried beans for 24 hours, changing the water frequently. Add baking soda to the water to neutralize the lectins further.

Removing these foods you're sensitive to completely for a short time can allow your gut to heal. Then reintroduce soaked beans and legumes and or sprouted wheat after the break. That can boost absorption of nutrients and reduce your sensitivity.

Beans are a good source of fiber and protein, so long as they are prepared correctly and you listen to your body. Not everyone will tolerate them even when you soak and sprout.

28. Test Yourself

I hint in many flips of food sensitivity. There are so many reasons why what you used to eat may not work to keep you feel good or looking great any more. Your gut health changes due to hormones, stress, and medications, and activity changes. The soil quality, the way foods are farmed, and the use of pesticides and fertilizers change the way we're influenced by food too. At any point you can become sensitive to foods you think of as "healthy."

The major triggers are wheat, gluten, dairy, eggs, soy, and peanuts, corn, and tree nuts. Food allergy labeling also includes fish and shellfish. If you have an autoimmune disease you also want to remove nightshade vegetables (tomatoes, peppers, eggplant). In the case of an allergy the immune system causes the symptoms of food intolerance. In non-allergenic food intolerance, a lack of enzymes does.

You may be thinking, what can I eat? You may not like me very much right now! While it can seem like you have to eliminate a lot of foods, you can make flips while you do it so there IS plenty you can eat. Flip from dairy milk to alternatives like almond, coconut, or hemp milk. Flip from wheat bread to brown rice tortillas or coconut wraps. There are flips for most everything.

Think of it as an adventure! What foods will you experiment with that you otherwise would not have? You may be amazed how much more energy you have to exercise and just live when you remove what's draining your body of energy.

It can be confusing and baffling to detect because food sensitivity can happen any time. You may have enjoyed milk and milk products your entire life and suddenly have symptoms like bloating, constipation, diarrhea, gas, or skin rashes. Less easy to detect are symptoms like fatigue, brain fog, weight gain/loss or inability to lose weight. Removing the high sensitive foods from your diet and reintroducing one by one can help pinpoint the foods that are problematic for you. Start today.

There's proof that overweight and obesity is caused in part by inflammation. Inflammation (caused by food sensitivity) can cause weight gain and the weight gain increases inflammation, making you further resistant to weight loss (in spite of exercise)! Temporary elimination followed by infrequent consumption of high sensitive foods can assist weight loss. In turn, weight loss further reduces inflammation. Win-win!

If you're nodding your head, yes, this makes sense, but you don't have any sense of urgency about changing, I invite you to do the 28-Day Kickstart. You'll be surrounded by other women on the same path and you will get it done and define your personal best foods to eat as you flip 50.

I'll share this best quote ever from a prior participant: I like feeling good!

Another said, "For me it was like trying on glasses. Until you put them on you have no idea what you're missing."

http://bit.ly/2xTVKv9

29. Get Gut Support

There are two things that can help you feel better, and want to move more.

First, digestive enzymes (Betaine HCL) help breakdown food and enhance micronutrient absorption. As we age, or stress, we don't breakdown proteins in food, as well. This will help. If you suffer from bloating and digestive issues, one possible cause is mal-absorption due to a lack of digestive enzymes.

People with Irritable Bowel Syndrome (IBS) get relief with digestive enzymes. During times of elevated stress, hormone changes, sleep disturbances, even if you aren't diagnosed with IBS, you too can benefit.

Second, a probiotic can help enhance your gut microbiome. That's code for the environment consisting of good and bad bacteria in the body. They become better balanced with support of probiotics. After a round of antibiotics or an illness it may be especially helpful to take probiotics through supplements to get them into the gut in a concentrated form.

You can follow that by getting probiotics through foods. Sauerkraut, kombucha, kimchi, and yogurt with live cultures added to your daily diet are ways to eat your probiotics. It just takes a few sips, spoon or forkfuls to keep your gut healthy.

Flipping 50 Fact: A specific gene might make a probiotics cause bloat due to an irritated gut lining. Adding digestive enzymes to your diet in that case may contribute to that bloating. About 20% of Caucasian adults fall into this category. If you experience bloating while taking probiotics and digestive enzymes, remove them for a week and see how you do. Check with a functional doctor for additional support.

30. Be Nice

Start talking to yourself more positively. Self-affirmations can help you change the story replaying in your head. Maybe you just need better communication skills, to use on yourself. If you want to make a change in some area of your life, whether it's food or exercise, and you want to either stop or start a habit, create a positive message around the change you want.

Instead of, I wish I could be more disciplined to exercise, say; I love the sense of accomplishment I have when I exercise.

Instead of, I wish I could be as good as _____ about sticking to my exercise plan, say, _____ is a great role model, and I'm going to set a regular routine for myself.

You also need to ask the right questions.

Instead of, why am I fat? Why can't I get motivated? or why don't I have any discipline? Ask first, do I want that to be true. Because in a way by asking that question you're stating that it's fact.

Then ask, what can I do today to take the best possible care of myself? What do I need to know or learn to get the results I want?

31. Train Fresh, Not Fatigued

Train most important muscles fresh, not when you're tired. Long distance runners... after a time running often begin to train incorrectly and default to lumber extension when they should be doing hip extension. You don't have to be a runner for this to have some relevance for you too. You too get tired and that's when you're most likely to train with poor form.

You want to train the good ones. Stop when form falls apart.

Let's take the core for example. We all need a strong core to do anything – daily activities require it. The stronger your core the easier you can lift more weight or go faster and therefore get better results.

Core-specific exercises are usually done at the end of an exercise session. There's a good reason. Your core should be fresh and able to stabilize during your exercise session. If core muscles are already fatigued, they may not do their job.

As you do perform those core exercises, it's important to think about how you train them. You either train for good form or you train for volume.

Especially if you have a history of low back pain you need to spend your exercise time training with perfect technique in a non-fatigued state. That is, do your most important core exercises when you're fresh.

Don't aspire to holding your plank for several minutes or beat someone's record on a YouTube video.

Renowned back care expert, Dr. Stuart McGill writes in his book Back Mechanic, you're better off doing multiple sets of shorter (10 second) prone and side bridges than you are trying to hold one set for 60 seconds. Train for a few minutes in the morning and at night instead of at a single longer session.

It's all about "turning on" the muscles from the off position. If you've ever experienced a surprising back injury this will make a lot of sense. You though perhaps you were strong, fit, and able to do your workouts just fine. Yet, during some fluke move you felt immediate pain. So you can hold a plank for 2 minutes. That doesn't insure that you can turn "on" the muscles well, since you've only rehearsed that once.

If you know the pain of injury to the low back, start with deep core stabilizers instead of flashy, circus act exercises. My Flat Abs Better Back DVD shows you how I recovered after a horseback riding accident years ago.

http://bit.ly/2kuS2m6

32. Pillow Talk

Assess your need for sleep. Do you:

- Plan to exercise in the morning but skip for a little more sleep?
- Wake up (sort of) not feeling rested?
- Yawn in the morning?
- Reach for caffeine and sugar?
- Have cravings get worse in the afternoon?

Get more sleep. That's the advice. It's easier said than done for way too many women in the middle of hormone changes. If you've changed your exercise, your diet, and you're working on your stress toolbox, without results, it's time to dial in your sleep. Sleep is mandatory for fitness results. Sleep is mandatory for maintaining lean muscle and losing fat.

The solution is not a nap. That's not why this flip is inserted in the middle of the book! A good night sleep takes some flips all day. Every exercise, nutrition, and daily flip you make can hurt or help your sleep. (It started with #1). If you choose this flip, you want to make sure you're ready tonight.

Add magnesium (to tolerance) to your evening meal to enhance your sleep.

Mary struggled with sleep when she started Flipping 50's 28-Day Kickstart. She didn't realize how much difference sleep would make on her weight loss success so she'd ignored poor sleep habits when she tried other diets and exercise programs.

She could go to sleep but then couldn't stay asleep or woke too early and then started her day groggy after hitting snooze too many times. Mary began taking magnesium at dinner and she was soon sleeping almost 2 hours more a night than her prior average. She was so thrilled with the way she felt the weight loss seemed less important. She ended up getting that too and lost 7-lbs during her 28 Day program.

A daily multivitamin usually contains the RDA 400 mg of magnesium. If you're taking a multi and still experiencing sleep challenges, doctor recommendations suggest to increase by taking 250 mg Magnesium Citrate with your evening meal for 3-5 nights. Magnesium deficiency is common. It's a "to-tolerance" micronutrient, so your best intake is unique to you.

See how you do and back off if you experience loose bowels or diarrhea. If you don't experience any benefit to sleep or any negative effects on digestion, increase to 500 and see how you do with that for another 3-5 nights. Continue with this process until you find the ideal for you.

Another way to boost magnesium and to relax before bed is soak in an Epsom salt bath about 90 minutes before bed. Your body will absorb what it needs and release the rest.

Flip tip: If you travel take along your magnesium supplement. Many of my functional health expert friends will boost their normal magnesium intake while traveling. Strange hotels, changing time zones, and dietary changes can wreak havoc on your system. Avoid sleep disturbances and constipation when you travel by packing magnesium.

Magnesium is responsible for so many enzymatic reactions in the body it may be a part of you sleeping, digesting, and having your metabolism work optimally.

Find out more about the importance of sleep and dozens of other ways to improve your pillow time (and reach optimal weight and energy) in Sleep Yourself Skinny.

http://bit.ly/2fIdzCv

33. Plug Your Leaks

Jump, lift, or bust a move in Zumba, then suddenly pee a little. Sound familiar? Low levels of the all-powerful sex hormones estrogen and testosterone can make it hard to make it through an exercise class without leaking. Up to 40% of women experience it. A lot lower percent every have a conversation with their doctor about what to do about it.

Exercise, at an intensity and type you're used to, does not in itself cause incontinence. Not even jumping and lifting actually cause the problem though they as well as sneezing and coughing can make you embarrassingly aware of it.

You can boost testosterone levels, or at least help them not plummet, by resistance training, performing short high intensity interval sessions, eating adequate protein and getting plenty of sleep. Avoid alcohol and sugar that sabotage your hormone levels.

Pelvic floor exercises, but not strength in general, do improve incontinence. Your vaginal muscles need a workout too. The fitness principle specificity applies to everything, right?

But there's more to it. And it's not surgery or expensive. Vaginal hormones can make a difference. Incontinence, prolapse, and sexual intimacy all stand to benefit with hormones inserted down there. Dr. Anna Cabeca's discovered that having patients apply testosterone and DHEA together down there resulted in so much success it ended her need to do surgical fixes. Through her research she developed a safe, non-surgical way to boost vag health that's tasteless, odorless and doesn't require an embarrassing conversation with your doctor to get it. She's been serving women for decades in private practice. There are other perks. I'll let you discover those for yourself.

If you want to take a quick quiz to learn more about your own incontinence, pelvic and sexual health confidentially visit Dr. Cabeca's site.

http://bit.ly/2wmESrO

34. Sip Bone Broth

It's still somewhat controversial if you Google it, but bone broth benefits include immunity boosting, and gut healing, and crave killing. Less research is available on the claims of weight loss, and collagen support for skin, hair, and nails. The benefit of using it as a nutrition upgrade for your broth in soups and stews is a significant increase in protein. Use it to cook your brown rice or quinoa.

The collagen protein found in bone broth is "better than Botox" say some! Collagen supports skin, connective tissue, joints and ligament health.

Sip it. If cravings derail you, digestive issues plague you, or you want to lose a few pounds without feeling deprived, bone broth could be your new BFF. I drink a cup or two daily and use it as the base in any soup or recipe calling for broth or water. If you're trying to avoid a snack habit a cup of bone broth offers about 8 grams of protein that just might do two things: keep you full and satisfied, and support recovery from exercise.

Though there is some controversy over whether the collagen boosting (think skintastic), gut healing benefits are proven in large studies, credible doctors sharing real results may sway you. A cup instead of your afternoon tea or coffee provides you with about 9 grams of protein. As an appetizer before lunch or dinner it can slow you down and so you eat more consciously. A fairly low sodium high protein bone broth drink may help you skip the colds this year by boosting your immune system.

In 1998 a study conducted at Iowa State University (go Cyclones!) found chicken soup is an effective recovery drink. Sans noodles, I'll have to agree and nod to my alma mater. Add some salt to the broth if you're using it for recovery from exercise and or as you nurse yourself back from the flu. The sodium is a part of the restoration of hydration and plasma volume.

I have skills but one of them is not making bone broth. I once bought all the ingredients and they spoiled before I got to it. I made it once, loved the way my house smelled but know my limits. I order mine from the bone broth authority, Kellyann Petrucci, The Bone Broth Dr., to be sure its made right and tastes great.

https://bv141.isrefer.com/go/cbbon112016/DebraAtkinson/

35. Stop the Processed

More than 10,000 chemicals are approved by the FDA for use in foods. It's a buyer beware world. Don't assume because it's in the health food section or a health food store, its green light go. A package is still a package. Fresh is best.

Many processed foods contain not just preservatives but artificial sweeteners. You may go sour on those sweet treats made with artificial sweeteners after reading this. They may be making or keeping you fat. The body responds to artificial sweeteners the same as it does to sugar. Blood sugar and insulin can spike and make fat storage more likely.

You're also conditioning your taste buds to want more sweet.

Like artificial sugar, your body responds poorly to anything chemical. If the body doesn't recognize it, it gets confused and slows your metabolism. If it preserves the shelf life of a food, it shortens yours.

I don't like rigid rules. Do you? One rule I do follow is eat as few bar codes as possible. If you're standing in your kitchen, why would you reach for a protein bar? Reach for nuts, seeds, or sun butter to put on an apple or celery stick.

"Which bar is best for traveling?" is a frequently asked question. If there is a bag of raw almonds, pistachios, or sunflower seeds beside the nut bars, go for the real food. In places you think you're limited by choices, there's usually a continuum of good, better, and best. Choose the best as often as you can.

36. Go Nuts for Another Butter

Flip your peanut butter passion to almond, cashew or sun butter. In fact, there are plenty of other nut butters to choose from. Peanuts are a common source of food sensitivity and maybe you've noticed, those who like their peanut butter usually like it a lot! The high mold in peanuts, and high allergen make this food less desirable than the other options available.

Flipping fit fact: If you're highly active and consuming peanuts or peanut products prior to exercise you may be more vulnerable to peanut-related sensitivity. During exercise you have increased absorption and could reach a threshold of allergic symptoms sooner. Trust me you don't want this to happen and you don't want it to happen to your jogging partner.

I used to jog with a friend in college. This was during the years when we thought salad bars were the panacea for health and we were body-conscious co-eds. It didn't take many afternoon jogs bringing on asthmatic symptoms a mile from our dorm for her to realize that she was sensitive to the preservative used to keep the greens greener on the cafeteria salad bar. While you might never have such an acute reaction spurred by exercise, you could still be experiencing the same internal inflammation.

If you're highly active and athletic you could naturally think that being more active and healthy you're less likely to be sensitive to foods. While you may absorb more nutrients too, you are more vulnerable to the bad stuff as well.

It's a good idea to keep your potential high sensitive food intake to an infrequent consumption whether you're highly active or not. During longer bouts of exercise choose carefully how to fuel before and during.

37. Be Back-Friendly

This goes for all exercises. It's normal to think about your back and core while you're doing back and core exercises. Sneaky little bad habits during other unsuspecting exercises can stress your back too.

Do you lock your knees when you're doing standing exercises? Do you arch your back when you raise a weight overhead?

You may not know the answers to those questions, yet. Start using a mirror while you're training and see what happens. It's easy to focus so much on the working muscles or be distracted that you forget the rest.

A few decades ago when I was just beginning to teach exercise we called this spatial awareness. It's important to think about each joint position to not only stay safe, but to get better results from exercise. You may be doing a triceps press for instance for those bat wings but you leverage the rest of your body while you're doing it.

Here are just a few tips for common exercises and the mistakes I most frequently see.

Bend your knees when you're doing any standing static exercise. Standing cable rows, bicep curls, triceps presses, and shoulder presses that you could do standing need slightly bent knees. Tip your pelvis very slightly forward if you have a curve in your low back. Just do this far enough to engage your core. If you're in the right spot you'll feel stronger and not as if you're in an awkward position.

Minimize stress on your back by using a split-stance on standing exercises like the bent over row. That means essentially, stand in a lunge position. It minimizes unwanted spine movement.

Know your limits. If you're doing standing exercises and catch yourself frequently locking your knees, sit. Bicep curls, triceps press, and bent over row for instance can all be done seated without reducing the benefit of the exercise. Performing exercises seated is appropriate whether you're just beginning or you're experienced and using a heavier weight than usual.

Hot, not hurt is your mantra.

38. Get a Better Butt

Who's in?

I'm not talking about the gravity slide that's causing body parts to rush to your socks. I'm not addressing the "Does my butt look big in these pants?"

But, or butt, those conditions might improve too.

Stronger gluteal muscles take a load off your spine. If you just suddenly thought of squats and lunges, that's logical, but they may not help. The small things matter most. If you have "gluteal amnesia" as many of us do thanks to sitting on our bums so many hours of the day, squats and lunges are not your go-to. Begin with isometric exercises. That's exercise with much less movement but very focused on isolating the lazy muscles. Here's your bun-lifting sequence.

1. Lie prone (belly down) on the floor with a pillow under your hips. Squeeze and release your gluteus on just one side 15 times. Repeat on the other.
2. To progress: Squeeze the gluteus on one side and then lift the leg a few inches. You shouldn't feel any pain in the lower back. Lower the leg to the floor and then release the gluteus. Repeat for a total of 15 times and then do a set on other leg.
3. Lie supine (on your back) on the floor. Bridge up so your knees, hips and shoulders are all in line. Hold for 5 seconds and release to the floor. Repeat 15 times.
4. Perform the previous exercise using just one side.

If in the middle of any of these exercises you feel you can't turn the muscles "on" any more, stop and rest, then start again. These muscles may essentially have ADD. As they get stronger with regular practice you'll be able to do more and fill your jeans in all the right places better too.

You can eventually add a second set to any of these exercises.

When you feel the contraction consistently you'll get more out of traditional leg presses, hamstring curls, squats and lunges if you're able to safely do those.

Buns up!

39. Pinpoint Pain

If you have back pain during certain abdominal exercises, stop doing them. Naturally, this seems obvious, but we've been conditioned to a "no pain no gain" approach.

The reality I recommend you adopt is, "no pain no gain: no brain." Pain is a message to your body that something is not right.

I've dwelled on stopping forward flexion exercises even if you don't feel pain elsewhere in this book. You can't always feel the progression to injury occurring. I'm about to sound very contradictory.

Pain is not always an indication there is risk of injury. Pain may not always be telling you the truth.

There is a time to work with bits of pain to bump a pain threshold. The key is in knowing when it's right to go there and override your brain and when to listen.

Liken the pain threshold to a beneficial stretch. When you stretch you want to go about 10% beyond the point where you feel resistance to the stretch. You hold in that slight discomfort to gradually increase your range of motion. While you hold a stretch the tension gradually eases. Stop and try it now. Breathe through a stretch and hold for 20-30 seconds.

So it is with getting to a new point of strength or function with an exercise when you've got some pain.

If you deal with chronic pain, this is naturally a scary step. Much of what you know about pain may be wrong. Pain originates in the brain rather than in the location in the body you feel the pain. By teaching the brain to respond differently you can begin to know the difference between good pain and bad pain. You can therefore train better and much more comfortably.

Dr. Joe Tatta, author of Heal Your Pain Now is a popular guest on the Flipping 50 podcast and is an expert on healing your pain. Learn more about healing your pain:

http://bit.ly/2k0X992

Part II

All Day Energy Flips

40. Heal Your Hunger

Your weight may not have anything to do with a lack of discipline or willpower. Starting a diet and exercise program may be like putting a band-aid on a broken leg.

Do you eat and eat without ever getting full? You feel uncomfortable and remorse about what you've done but you're never satisfied. Is that you?

Don't misunderstand. Exercise is a significant predictor of long-term weight loss. It is far less tied to energy expenditure than you might think, however. At some point you will need to know the right things to put in your body. You'll need to know the right exercise for your needs. But first there could be something far more beneficial.

Emotional eating (EE) is different than not knowing what to eat. Having a perfect diet won't fix it. Exercising regularly won't make EE go away. It's a unique challenge that requires a unique solution.

There's no skirting around the fact we have to have some kind of relationship with food. We tie emotions to food through the dash from birth to death. If you're an emotional eater, healing is about more than changing what you eat, how you exercise, or your weight.

If you:

- Restrict food
- Binge eat

- Purge
- Constantly diet
- Obsess about food
- Exercise to exhaustion

Then I encourage you to seek support from a friend of mine. Tricia Greaves Nelson has been there. She's 50 and she gets you too. Her book and program Heal Your Hunger are a best first step to heal. Get to the root of emotional eating for insights, answers, and a better way to deal with emotions.

http://bit.ly/2y12vLL

42. Go Green

You know when things sometimes sound too good to be true? How would you like to burn 29% more fat after your workout?

It's good.

It's true.

Add Matcha to a smoothie 60-90 minutes before an interval training session. This green tea extract can improve fat oxidation that occurs after intervals by 29%.

If you can manage it with your schedule this timing is perfect for a pre-exercise protein shake. Add matcha to your green smoothie in the morning before intervals 1-2 times a week for a fat burning boost. The research is done with intervals and subjects were post-menopausal. So you know it has the potential to help you!

There's good reason to believe that with high force strength training to fatigue the increase in fat oxidation would also be true. So get into a habit of doing that pre-exercise matcha boost before any intense exercise. Make it a simple latte with hot, not boiling, almond milk and matcha, sweetened with a bit of matcha if a smoothie is too much before exercise.

Take the flip further: even resting values of fat oxidation increased by 24%. So yes, if you're wondering if you can do it after instead of before, or if adding matcha on your rest days or recovery exercise days is also a good idea? Flipping, yes! Keep in mind, Matcha with caffeine provided the fat burning boost while caffeine-free did not. Keep your matcha intake to early in the day if you're sensitive to caffeine (and you want your high intensity exercise early anyway!)

Matcha also helped overall and abdominal fat loss with moderate exercise. So if you're limited by constrictions, or know yourself so well that intervals might prevent you from falling in love with exercise, start with the level of exercise you'll do and you'll still see some benefit with the addition of matcha.

Matcha has such a mild flavor that if you have a sensitive palate you may have to get used to it but it's not bitter and if you have flavorful protein shake mix and some fruit added you may not even notice it except for the green color it's going to give your smoothie.

Is consuming matcha better than sipping your green tea for fat burning? Studies say yes. In supplemental form (the powdered green tea extract), matcha, provides benefits in a serving size equivalent to 8-10 cups of tea a day and offers better results.

The Tea Spot founder (and MIT mechanical engineer), Maria Uspenski shared as guest on Flipping 50 that 5 cups of tea a day significantly decrease your risk of several cancers according to the National Institute of Health. With one shot of Matcha you're well on your way to immediate gratification and long-term health benefits.

42. Eat for Sleep

Nine out of ten women who begin a Flipping 50 program have two things in common.

They have severely reduced carbohydrate consumption at night.

Their rating of sleep quality is 5/10 or less.

That's not coincidence. If you are struggling to sleep and lose weight both, there's a chance that the very thing you're doing to reach your weight loss goal is sabotaging both that and short-sheeting you on sleep.

Carbohydrates boost your natural production of serotonin. Serotonin is your feel-good hormone. Women have lower levels of it than men. Too little of it can make you feel depressed. The right amount helps keep you calm and will improve your readiness to sleep in the evening.

Though simple math about carbohydrate storage in the body can make you lose weight quickly by removing carbohydrates it could sabotage you later. For every one-part carbohydrate stored, three parts water is stored. Eliminate carbs and you'll lose water weight. After a short time, driving your carb intake too low can disrupt your sleep and cause cravings you can't out-willpower.

Dinnertime is a good time to eat more carbohydrates. That is, eat more than you have at previous meals in the day.

Still with me?

I know it's often the exact opposite of what you may be doing. But if you're both sleepless and weight loss has stalled, what have you got to lose? Women usually come back within a week and tell me they can't believe how much more energy they have, and how much happier they are! We do love our carbs. The trick is to not go for the breadbasket or the chips to do it.

Try one or two of these suggestions for a full week and see what happens.

Tonight, have a sweet potato with your dinner. If you prefer, have some brown rice or quinoa. Make a butternut squash soup or have chili made with means. Finish with a small cup of berries.

43. Go Fish

Eating more fish could decrease your risk of obesity and metabolic syndrome. If you know you should be eating more fish, make sure you know the safety of the fish you're eating. Unfortunately, our waters are so contaminated with chemicals that almost all of the largest fish are toxic and carry risk of mercury. Tuna, halibut, and salmon all so often promoted as good sources of Omega 3 fat require a second look.

If you consume a lot of fish or rely on canned or bagged big fishes for your pantry, check labels carefully. Smaller fish are less toxic. Try making your old favorite tuna salad with sardines as a healthier substitute.

Heavy metals can accumulate in the body. When they do your body can't function correctly. Metal toxicity depends on how much you absorb, and whether it was acute or chronic exposure. Chronic fatigue can be one risk of exposure to heavy metals. Blood tests specifically for heavy metals can reveal whether this is a problem for you.

Most of the warnings about mercury levels in fish still target pregnant women, those wanting to become pregnant, and children. Yet, the longer we live in a world exposed to toxins, and endocrine hormone disrupters, the more careful you want to be so you can protect our health.

Fish are a big source of mercury, but other 22 other heavy metals including arsenic, cadmium, chromium, copper, lead, nickel, and zinc pose a threat to health. Exposure comes from soil erosion, pesticides on crops for insect control, and from diet.

Everything you drink, eat, and breathe has the ability to make you healthier or inhibit your best health. Heavy metals can interfere with hormone balance and ultimately hormone affects metabolism. So if you're struggling to lose weight and you've adopted proper hormone balancing exercise and changed your diet to support it, consider asking your physician about a specific heavy metal blood test to determine if this could be a problem for you.

44. Double Down

Double your resistance training volume. That is, if it's appropriate for you. Those who can do more in this case should. That means if you're healthy with no special conditions – you may want to bump your three sets to six. That's a big bump so see below for more details.

A study has shown that with older adults who are most at risk for losing lean muscle, increasing the volume of resistance training exercise increases muscle protein synthesis (MPS).

Muscle protein synthesis decreases with age, but both increasing protein intake following exercise, and increasing the volume of resistance training significantly increased MPS in subjects whose average age was 70.

If you're an older adult thinking you should slow down, or wondering if it's wise do more at your age, the answer, is clearly yes. If you want to be stronger, full of energy, stamina and strength for living you can exercise your way there. If you have a special condition limiting you, of course you'll need to pay attention to that. Just don't let your mind be what limits you.

If you're considering doubling your sets use a smart progression. Add a set this week, another next, constantly assessing for pain or more soreness than usual. If you lift twice a week, try increasing volume just one day a week for a month or two.

Older women, compared with older men, have a blunted anabolic response to both eating and exercise and may therefore need more of both protein and resistance training to achieve the same gains in lean muscle as seen in men.

You may not want to be so quick to take the smaller portion of protein you're serving up tonight. Take the big one for yourself.

45. Scoop on Your Poop

The quality of your poop will tell you about the quality of your diet and your gut health. Are you pooping rocks, snakes, or pudding? Your goal is snakes. Rocks tell you that you need more water and more fiber by increasing your vegetables and fruit intake. Pudding tells you that you need to reduce your fiber.

If you aren't processing food correctly inside it will be hard to see the results from exercise on the outside. A lack of exercise results may have less to do with your sets and repetitions and more to do with your digestion.

If you've been putting up with constipation, diarrhea, gas, bloating and just passing it off (pun intended) as normal for you, don't! These things aren't normal, they're just signs. Adjust your diet to improve your gut health by eliminating foods that trigger these issues so you can fix your gut lining. It will make everything more enjoyable.

If you've got a fear of eliminating foods you love forever, that is not usually necessary. There may be something you can't have all the time. But most things you'll be able to have some of the time as long as you let your gut heal first.

It's time to eliminate (I couldn't help myself) embarrassing or uncomfortable exercise or the need to stay close the toilet.

46. Herb Your Hormones

Consider herbs for a natural approach to some of your nagging hormone problems and to boost your exercise performance. If you're currently taking a prescription medication or bioidentical hormones, ask your practitioner before you start to be sure there are no negative interactions. Ashwaganda, maca, and rhodiola are three herbs that may help with hot flashes, energy, and night sweats.

Maca is a hormone-balancing adaptogen. It helps reduce cortisol and boost libido. Its self-regulating meaning if you need it you'll get it, if you don't you won't. You'll find it in the health food section and you can easily add it to smoothies. My favorite way to add maca is to a cherry vanilla smoothie post-exercise.

Rhodiola is another adaptogen, with the ability to balance hormones in non-specific situations so that essentially, if you need it, it will help you adapt to stressors by decreasing cortisol levels and enhancing energy and endurance.

Ashwatanga helps your tolerance to stress by lowering cortisol levels and may help with hot flashes and night sweats. It is associated with better performance in athletes, potentially because of its cortisol lowering capability.

47. Take Three Polite Bites

Three polite-sized bites of any one food are not going to destroy what you do most of the time. You will enjoy the taste and remove power from any food. Once you allow yourself to have it, you may just choose not to do so. This freedom gives you back a lot of energy and time spent thinking about foods you have not let yourself have.

There are two things that make this flip work. First, your taste buds turn over in about 11 days. That means you may have to operate on a little willpower or discipline and avoid those sweet treats for that amount of time. Then if there's a sweet you're subjected to, try it. Savor it. You may find that those three bites are plenty because you're so much more sensitive to sweet.

Second, don't allow food to have power over you. If bringing a chocolate bar into the house is too much temptation for you, don't. Make yourself have to make multiple decisions about eating it. You're better off having to get in the car, go to the store or restaurant, order one serving, and enjoy it rather than bringing it into your home. You may plan to have just one little square after dinner but if that repeatedly turns into the whole bar, why would you do that to yourself?

I live close to three of the sweetest great-nephews on the planet. Their mom is a rock star at creating themed birthday cakes for them. I usually enjoy a big corner piece (that's where the frosting is) and sometimes I even eat the cake. By the time I put my fork down, it keeps me for another few months 'til the next birthday.

There's no regret. There's no punishing exercise to "burn it off." It doesn't work that way, anyway. Your body naturally turns up the thermostat and burns off the occasional extras as long as you usually do the right thing. You'll love the next flip!

48. Be Consistent, Not Perfect

"The more consistent you are, the less perfect you have to be."

This quote from 1972 Olympic marathon winner Frank Shorter is a gem. This is true in your exercise plan, your nutrition, and your sleep.

Frank meant it in reference to the way he trained for that first marathon in Olympic history that he had decided should be run more like a track race than a slog (slow jog). He changed the history of marathon competition by doing that. He didn't do it by running fast all the time.

He trained mostly for the foundation of fitness that would allow him to run it faster. The majority of his training time was spent building that fitness level to build everything else on.

Assess yourself today.

Are you exercising consistently? Are you consistently eating the things that your body thrives on? It's easy to fall into the trap of thinking about it more frequently than you actually do it. It's so easy to say, this week is hard, I'm busy, I have company, I _____________ (fill in the blank). If you get to the end of too many weeks having done this, you're consistently ditching the most important part of your fitness plan.

Consistency is your best friend. During a busy day, movement may have to happen in 10 minutes instead of that half hour. It may happen at home instead of at the gym. It may be that you have to take a few short cuts to get the veggies and lean protein and healthy fats at the store instead of preparing them from scratch. Yet, making these choices is what makes you the winner at the finish.

Your second best friend is intensity. A yearlong study showed that consistent exercise in a supervised program for 6 months improved strength, body composition, and wellbeing in older adults. But after subjects either continued on their own or stopped, six months after the study, there was no significant difference in either group. You have to be doing something worthwhile consistently.

Take out your calendar and add the workouts and the time you may need to spend preparing for meals. Make yourself first. If you begin to do this and it's a mystery for you exactly what is the thing to do, ask! Get a workout partner, a trainer, or an online group. Find a community that holds you accountable to more than you will do on your own. Beginners and elite athletes both know they need coaches. In the middle of that continuum is ego telling you that you ought to be able to do it on your own or you are so disciplined or motivated that you don't need help.

Ride your bike with someone who is faster. Run with someone with more endurance. Train with someone who is using heavier weight. Who are you going to do your workouts with?

49. Take Responsibility

Stop thinking it is anyone else's job to determine what you eat and when. Start planning ahead. Ask for what you need. It's OK to be high maintenance. Right now while the resistance is great, and 80% of US population is not exercising enough to benefit health and obesity is still high, it's normal to feel if you care for yourself you're swimming upstream. Expect resistance. You'll be ready.

If eating certain foods or ingredients were life threatening for you, you would do what you needed to do. Your life will indeed be compromised if you eat foods that don't serve you well. Nearly any restaurant anywhere can accommodate someone with known food-allergies. If that's true, they can accommodate you and your food preferences. Ask for what you want and need. Menus are, in fact, a suggestion. It is your choice.

Go ahead and be that girl. You know the one I mean. The one who does her thing instead of succumbing to peer pressure when others are not on the same path. She's not judging others, she's just making sure she feels her best today and tomorrow and the next day.

You can live for the moment. But if you're hating the little voice in your head, don't like your energy level, or feel like the reflection in the mirror isn't reflecting the radiant you that it could be? Flip it.

This isn't about skipping the party or not going out, unless you really don't want to. It's about knowing it's OK to tell the hostess that you can't eat dairy or soy or that you're avoiding sugar and gluten. It's about asking if you can bring something to make it easy for her (and you). It's about you saying, "something dairy-free, soy-free, and nut free salad" when someone asks if they can bring something.

No one you know wants to wake up feeling like crap. Do you remember ever thinking that would be fun? Food made without the most common high sensitive foods is delicious, just different than what you may be used to, and doesn't come with the upset stomach, or bloat. That's a truly generous hostess or guest.

I have a friend who travels frequently for speaking engagements. She makes veggies ahead of time, brings them in insulated containers and coolers on planes, trains, and automobiles. She's been sick. Now she's well and she's not giving it up. She'll be in an airport eating her home-prepared meals while others are picking over expired salads with preservatives on them. You would never know she's on the road half of every week. Her skin is radiant. Her form is lean. Her energy is sky high. It can be done. It's just like packing shoes for her. It's not optional.

Community helps. If you need someone to tell you "just keep swimming" regularly, join a group who will do that. Flipping 50's members-only Café is such a community dedicated to women over 50.

http://bit.ly/2y7BLGZ

50. Get Hot Not Flashy

Exercise improves bone density, decreases risk of depression, and improves body composition. All that is fine and dandy, but if you're in the middle of a hot flash, you're not so motivated to further increase your sweat rate or risk bringing another one on. You want to know the answer to one question.

Will exercise decrease hot flashes?

Yes.

Reduce your hot flash frequently with exercise. Increase hot flash frequency (by 28%) with couch time. It's been proven that with both continuous moderate, and high intensity interval training, as well as resistance training, there are improvements directly related to hot flashes.

A 16-week exercise training intervention significantly reduced hot flash weekly frequency by approximately 62%.

Exercise helps you regular body heat better overall. In doing that, hot flashes are reduced in frequency or intensity.

How much exercise does it take to get you hot, not bothered?

Thirty minutes three times a week. Start there.

Increase your duration and frequency gradually to 45 minutes 4 or 5 times a week.

Yes, provided it's of adequate intensity. So your hot flash-specific workout can follow the same drill you would for getting hot.

Say yes to interval training one or two times a week, a steady state session one or two times a week, and pull in a couple resistance training sessions a week.

Hello hot.

51. Make It Stick

"I fell off the wagon and got ran over by it."

That is not my favorite way to start a coaching call with a client.

But it happens. __it happens.

To help habits stick when it all hits the fan, prepare for it. The biggest problem with goal setting is that we fail to prepare for the obstacles. It all starts in honeymoon phase. It never stays there.

If you don't create a list of solutions for dealing with potential interruptions, they'll win.

Before you adapt a new habit or goal or if you're trying to get back on track with one, answer these:

- How are you going to benefit?
- How will you suffer if you don't change?
- Who else will benefit if you change?
- Who will it hurt if you don't change?
- What could get in the way?
- How will you stay on track when that happens?

None of those questions remove the likelihood stressful things will interrupt you but you should have a clear idea of how important (or not) this goal is to you.

People who adhere to regular exercise have usually shifted from having to remember to do it or trying to fit it in to a place where it's just a part of them and what makes them feel best. Before you get there, it takes conscious planning.

Plan A: Develop your best plan.

Plan B: Create a second best.

Plan C: Identify an if-all-else-fails backup.

A flexible plan keeps you consistent. Do this for your exercise, diet, and any daily habits that you're trying to adapt. Focus on them one-by-one.

Carrie went through my Kickstart program. She wanted to lose weight but felt it was impossible due to her work schedule. She traveled at least 3 days a week. Her cross-country commute had her up too early to exercise and still in meetings too late at night to exercise two days of her workweek. Food was provided at meetings and she didn't have any choice in options. She ended up feeling "hung over" after every trip that lost her even more days.

Self-affirmations come in handy in situations like this. But first, you have to address limiting beliefs. To identify Carrie's limiting beliefs I asked her:

- How much time do you think it takes?
- Does 10 minutes serve you better than nothing?
- What foods could you carry with you?
- Do you have to eat when you're at a meeting?
- Can you make a special request?

She started using these affirmations:

- 10 minutes of exercise gives me energy all day
- I feel so much better when I eat the right foods and avoid the wrong ones.

You can be successful under stress.

52. Brace Yourself

Stop trying to "draw your navel to your spine." Ignore instructions to "suck in your belly button." These cues refer to "hollowing."

Toss out hollowing in favor of bracing.

Hollowing actually weakens your core muscles. It interferes with their ability to perform. Instead you want to stiffen the muscles.

Many exercises you've probably have already adopted are bracing. Planks, for instance, or pushups and bridges naturally encourage bracing. Have you ever tried to suck your belly button to your spine while doing one of those? You can't, or you can't do the exercise.

If I throw a ball to you, naturally you brace. I don't need to cue you to do it. When a small child hurls him or herself toward you the same thing happens. Bracing is life. Hollowing is trying to squeeze into too tight pants for a second, button them up, and then let go only to be miserable as long as you have them on. It isn't sustainable.

You might be told in a fitness class to hollow or suck the belly button in while you do a rocking motion through the pelvis to enhance mobility. That makes sense. Just don't try to make a muscle stronger by putting it in a weakened condition. That sentence doesn't even make sense, so why would core exercise like that make sense?

Planks and pushups are static bracing. Life, you may have noticed, is pretty dynamic. You don't have to have a ball thrown at you to practice dynamic bracing. You can throw a ball at a wall or bounce it as hard as you can on the ground, standing on one or two feet.

Train for life. Life is constantly getting things thrown at you, literally and figuratively.

Brace yourself.

53. Build Brain Health

Mindful workout planning can build your brain as much as your body. A workout that allows your brain to wander won't do it but an interval-training workout or a new weight workout that requires you to focus on form while you get an intense workout will.

Does that mean that your leisure walk around the neighborhood isn't helping your health? It is. But it's not helping your brain as directly. You'll reduce your perceived stress levels and support hormone balancing with that stroll. However, high intensity exercise efforts that make you to monitor your body response to effort and keep track of time requires focus that heightens your brain benefits.

Interval training sessions can be done by anyone. High intensity exercise doesn't have to be high impact. Water exercise, cycling, rowing, or boxing intervals provide lower impact options.

In fact, it's possible to improve fitness – and brain health - as you age, even after you turn 100, according to a study in the Journal of Applied Physiology.

Make your next workout one that makes you pay attention. Your brain and your body will both thank you.

54. Calm Yourself

Get hot not bothered. Women with higher levels of anxiety have greater incidence of hot flashes. There's another reason to love resistance training. Besides the muscle that will boost metabolism, the bone density, the look-good-naked component, and a dozen other reasons to fall in love with weight training, studies show it also decreases anxiety levels.

You're not your mother, sister, or bestie so you may have to find your own ideal way to lift weights. Whether it's alone in your living room, at a class, or solo in the weight room at the gym, resistance training can reduce the intensity of hot flashes.

One warning, if you're just starting out have patience. As you elevate your core temperature during a workout it may at first trigger a hot flash. Stick with it and as you increase your fitness level and well being, anxiety levels will drop and you'll be able to benchmark less severe flashes. All that's left, then will just be hot you.

If you love yoga, wonderful, do yoga. It too reduces stress, and increases cognitive function (goodbye brain fog, hello again memory). If you have a limited amount of time however, knowing every exercise is mind-body is freeing! You don't have to make exercise a part or full time job. You don't have to spend hours a day at the gym to look and feel good.

The most important foundation for getting benefits is choosing something you love. Stop questioning whether it's the perfect exercise. Start asking, is this perfect for me?

55. Skip the Scale

Get ready for a shocker.

Even if the first goal you have is to lose weight, it won't be the thing that motivates you most. This was true for subjects in a study whether they were normal weight, overweight, or obese. Weight loss was just too broad to target daily habits.

Focus on habits that improve your blood pressure, cholesterol, and blood sugars. You'll live longer and better, potentially more than simply being "thin or slimmer."

The bonus if you do have weight to lose? If your habits improve those health measures, your body will also release extra weight because you've balanced your hormones. You can have what you ultimately want. You just have to go about getting it with a different approach.

You can have a body you love after 50. Just as long as you don't try to get it using things that worked at 30.

In 34 years I can't think of a single woman whose goal was a certain size and weight who ever relaxed once she got there. Losing weight to reach a certain size comes with a fear of keeping the weight off and constant thinking about it, and talking about it.

That's a vicious cycle.

If you live with constant thoughts about food, exercise, and weight, it's not your fault. The message is everywhere encouraging you to think this way. The media, your Facebook page, even other female friends who are critical of their own bodies or who are always on a diet play right into that message that if you're not the air-brushed image yet you should be on your way.

When those thoughts bring you to the scale to tell you if you're happy today or not, something is wrong. This brings to mind conversations I have too frequently with clients. During a coaching call early in our relationship my client Melinda shared that she was already experiencing so much more energy, she was sleeping better, and her bloating was gone. Her voice was full of energy and high pitched with excitement.

Then, she said this, "So I was sure that I must have lost weight but when I got on the scale nothing had changed." Her voice was suddenly low and slow, void of energy and enthusiasm.

Have you done this? You feel amazing, and you've got evidence that what you're doing is working and yet, you give up all your power to the scale. You think if the scale doesn't say it's true then it's not true.

It's time to kick that those thoughts (and your scale) to the curb.

If you do lose weight you have no idea if you're losing fat (or muscle) unless you're tracking that too. You can get a body composition test done in minutes at any fitness center. If you ever buy another scale make sure it has a body composition-tracking feature.

If body composition testing isn't available or you feel too embarrassed to go get it done, at least track your measurements along with weighing so you'll have plenty of evidence. Try on several pair of pants while you're at it. Your inches will change much more quickly than your weight if you are losing body fat and gaining lean muscle. Your proportions may change (for the better) or you could reduce inches all over.

You'll control the shape of things most if you're weight training. (Cardio queens beware: you'll have the same body shape issues just smaller without weight training. If you want to be the boss of your body shape pick up the weights.) If you have more weight to lose your inches will change more noticeably at first and then slow but they will continue to change if you have weight to release.

You may be like my client Martina. She keeps reporting another slow loss of a pound or two at each of our calls. But the pants she couldn't wear last spring fell to the floor when she put them on in the early fall.

That works.

56. Support Sleep

Is it time to pull out the heavy artillery?

If you've tried everything, consistently, and haven't found anything that works to improve your sleep, consider melatonin.

Try melatonin 90 minutes before bed. Your body produces less of it as you age. It's a hormone with few negative side effects, though some women do report feeling groggy the morning after taking it. This may be due to the type of melatonin taken. Some melatonin supplements are released immediately and some are more time-released. If you take a time-released option to help you stay asleep and avoid those nasty 2am stair-at-the-ceiling wake ups, but if you don't take it early enough it may be still in your system in the morning.

Test yourself and your tolerance to melatonin to see if it's helpful for you. Most commonly, 3 grams is a starting point. Test several nights in a row consistently to determine if your sleep is supported by melatonin. Testing requires making one change at a time, so be sure you keep a consistent bedtime routine and don't make other changes while you're testing this one. Most of the women in Flipping 50's 28 Day Kickstart who opt for melatonin benefit from taking it 90 minutes before bed so it's get it can work it's magic by bedtime.

Don't rely on any pill to do the work of good sleep habits. Set a bedtime that gives you adequate sleep considering your wake time. Start winding down 90 minutes before that. Get into a routine that works for you. Good suggestions include shutting off screens, reading a book, taking a bath or shower. See more details in Sleep Yourself Skinny.

http://bit.ly/2fIdzCv

Track your results with a simple sleep journal every morning.

57. Tone with Testosterone

Are you strength training without results? Do you feel like you're losing tone every day?

Your testosterone may need a boost. This hormone we associate more with men is an important one for your lean muscle. You have less of it to begin with and even that amount can begin to dwindle.

Start these testosterone-enhancing habits:

- "Sprint" or try High Intensity Intervals 1-2 times a week
- Weight train with fewer repetitions and heavier weight
- Take longer rest periods between sets
- Fuel for your workout (and life) with adequate calories and protein
- Get plenty of sleep
- Decrease stress and anxiety

Avoid these testosterone-depleting habits:

- Sugar
- Alcohol
- Too much long slow exercise
- Absence of weight training
- Skipping meals or protein (listen to the recordings in your book bonuses)
- Burning the candle on both ends

The very thing you used to do to lose weight gets in the way of you having more lean muscle tissue and balanced hormones. That's going to increase your fat. Old habits may be already catching up with you. In midlife all those little mistakes we've made are amplified.

Eat more of the right foods, exercise less, and with purpose and you'll support more optimal testosterone.

If you need added incentive, the next flip might do it.

58. Boost Your libido

I get letters for the Flipping 50 TV show from women who write, My husband and I used to be adventurous and had a great sex life, but lately my libido needle is bouncing on empty. It's not fair to him or to me. What can I do?

The same thing that reduces your ability to see toned muscles from exercise and causes more of the fat in places you don't want it is responsible. Testosterone strikes again. So review flip #57 and dial up your results to avoid tanking testosterone.

If you're overdoing exercise to get extra weight off you may be draining yourself and have nothing left over for the bedroom. Stay focused on the hard-to-accept fact that short bouts of exercise increase your energy level while long ones can drain you. (Long ones can also increase your appetite and backfire by sending you snacking or making you cranky if you don't give in.)

The right kind of exercise (flip #57) will give you more body confidence. Women with a low libido often tell me that they don't like the way they look and they don't want their partner's hands touching them.

Just a gentle reminder that usually in the room with a naked partner, it probably matters a whole lot less to your significant other! But that doesn't change the way you feel and that's what's important.

Weight training and a regular high quality whole food diet that includes adequate protein, fat, fiber, and antioxidants are your best allies for a hot, not bothered body.

There are intangible things you need to handle, too. Stress kills libido. Stressors aren't going anywhere, so this is about handling it better. You need a bring-it-on attitude. Add joy to your life. If you've declared war on carbs, try adding a few back in to boost your serotonin levels. The right carbs at the right time help you reduce anxiety and stay calm. That makes it more likely to rev up.

Be sure when you are in bed not operating that libido you're getting sleep! Overtired and wired, it would be impossible for a woman at any age to be in the mood. You support lower stress with sleep. Even if you aren't emotionally stressed, without adequate sleep your cortisol levels are not going to support romance. Read flips #32, #42, and #56 for more on sleep strategies.

The combination of building body confidence with the right weight training and supporting nutrition together with small stress-reducing habits every day (give each other a hug, laugh – at anything, add 3 things to a gratitude list) can bring back or enhance your libido.

Do you have a question for Flipping 50 TV? Send it to me at Flipping50TV.com and if I choose your question for the show you'll get some gifts from our sponsors and me. https://www.flippingfifty.com/flipping-50-tv/

Are you watching? The shows are posted at flippingfifty.com under the Flipping 50 TV tab. Please share the show with a friend!

http://bit.ly/2yxNVvV

59. Exercise Caution

Avoid exercise dependence.

This may seem like odd advice coming from a fitness professional. I've seen women in midlife become dependent on exercise for their sense of well-being. It's their first defense against stress. That's both good and bad.

If you've lived a good life, and had a little fun along the way, you have your share of small aches and pains, or "limiters," as I call them. Overreliance on exercise for stress reduction can lead to increased risk of injuries. You have less resilient joints, ligaments, and muscles. Make no mistake I'm not saying you should slow down. You just want a mindful balance between work and rest to be your best body.

When life drops stressors on you and you're exercise dependent, your response is probably to exercise more. Unless, say the stressor is a physical injury, and then you're a basket case because you don't have a release for your stress. (It takes a basket case to know a basket case.)

The fact is that exercising more during emotional stress can quickly lead to a physical injury. Your body deals with all stress the same. So at some point, enough will be enough.

I've had my share of overreliance on exercise to negate stress. During grad school I was teaching a multiple fitness classes daily and then doing my own workouts on top of it. I was definitely more tired than better. Still, that was my feel-good fix. Send the endorphins in to help me cope with statistics and chemistry, please!

More recently, I was training for an endurance event. The same year I'd gone through about eight life stressors I don't recall putting my hand up for. Though I love the plan and purpose in training for an event, suddenly just a few weeks before the race a 5-year-old injury reared its ugly head.

It's like my body said, "Enough. If you don't get that this is too much to deal with at one time, I'll show you what I mean." I did the event – scared- in a very compromised way to reduce further stress. Immediately, after the event, and I mean hours, the injury disappeared. I was lucky there was nothing more serious. You have to know the signs and symptoms of "too much" for you.

Take some time when life is in flow for you and stress is low to develop ways other than exercise for coping. For women, venting helps. Call a friend. Get outdoors. Laughter can do wonders. Maybe for you it's a book, a movie, or a scroll through your Facebook page for a funny.

Healthy coping mechanisms are the goal. A glass of wine, maybe. A bottle? Not so much. If the physical purge still appeals to you most fill what would be exercise time with a massage, a hot tub soak or sauna time.

60. Core More Often

More core exercise frequency is better than longer duration. If you have little endurance for back exercises, it's best to do repeats of short duration. Hold 10 seconds in a plank and repeat 6 times, for instance, instead of attempting to hold for 60 seconds. At point you'll be ready to progress. Avoid the natural urge to just add time.

Once you're doing longer repetitions of planks, hold the longest first, and decrease the hold time with repeats. Hold the first one 1:00, rest and hold the second 45 seconds, rest and plank 30 seconds, rest and so on.

"Dumb" or lazy muscles have a short attention span! Whether you're starting, restarting, or beginning core exercise after an injury, instead of doing an exercise three times a week for 20 minutes, do it three times a day for 5. Gradually, you can progress to a single session a day as your tolerance for exercise increases.

Here's a sample progression.

Start:

- 2-3 10-second plank repeats
- 2-3 5-second bridge repeats
- 3 times a day

Progress:

- 2-3 20-second plank repeats
- 5 5-second bridge repeats
- 3 times a day

Progress:

- 1 each 30-second/20-second/10 second plank repeats
- 10 bridges
- 2 times a day

Progress:

- 1 each 45-second/30-second/20-second plank repeats
- 15 bridges
- 2 times a day

Progress:

- 1 each 1-minute/45-sec/30-sec/15 sec plank
- 12 5-second bridges
- 1 time a day most days of the week

Report your progress or share your question on the Flipping 50 community page on Facebook.

https://www.facebook.com/flipping50tv

61. Fake Change

The placebo effect can improve your health.

Think about the times you've been sick and have paid big bucks for a "horse pill." Scientists find it's not just the pill, but taking the pill thinking that it will make you well, makes you well.

It works even if you know you're doing it. You can prepare your brain for healing, or for improved energy or sleep.

Taking a magnesium supplement with dinner may in fact help you relax and sleep better. But believing it will, can enhance the probability more. So much so that if you stop taking it might make you believe that you will lose sleep.

As I write, this exact thing happened to me last night. Before I went to sleep I realized that I'd forgotten to take my melatonin. I didn't want to get up again. I thought to myself, great, I need a good night sleep!

Sure enough, 2:30am found me unable to go back to sleep. I'm a good sleeper! This does not happen to me! I'm convinced it was the thought, not the lack of the pill that did it. The week before while traveling I'd forgotten to pack the bottle. I slept like a rock.

Studies are showing that it doesn't matter whether you take (and know it is) a placebo or a real pill during medical trials. The ritual and focus on the healing process may be a part of the success of placebo, as might any additional attention or outside focus and attention.

Pay attention to what you want. Create an expectation for results. If your mindset shifts so you believe actions you're taking will help, they will.

Click your shoes, Dorothy, and while you're at it, state the outcome you want.

Remember The Secret? The book and documentary featured a form of placebo effect. The Law of Attraction is closely related to your intentions and your belief that you can bring the desired outcomes you want into your life. The mixed reactions and stir among professionals about The Secret came because there wasn't enough emphasis on taking action after declaring what you want.

Yes, declare your desire. Then go get it with a clear set of actions.

You need to wish for it, AND work for it.

You may or may not need to believe it. There have been results proving the effectiveness of a placebo even with non-believers.

62. Work In

You don't have to lose your memory.

Strong focus to the point your brain gets tired strengthens your cortex.

A Harvard Medical School study found adults over 60 that have memories as good or better than 18-to-32-years old have kept their cortex from thinning. They've done it by stimulating their brains with intensity. The same rules that apply to exercise workouts apply to your brain.

Force yourself to focus on hard tasks. Learning a new language and playing games that challenge you are good, word searches aren't.

Combine your exercise and learning sessions to enhance both your brain and body. While you're doing any exercise, focus on the muscle fibers, identify the name of the muscle, think about where it begins (origin) and ends (insertion). Do a little research or have your trainer quiz you.

When you perform resistance exercise with power (speed during the lift), mentally list the benefits of doing power. Count your repetitions in another language. Once you've mastered one new language move on to another. Then challenge yourself: first set Spanish, second set German, and so on.

We often dissociate (distract ourselves with TV, a magazine, or music) instead of associate (connect to the details) while we exercise. Enhance your benefits by connecting your brain and your body.

Ironically, thinking about nothing also helps your cortex. Meditation is rapidly becoming mainstream. You don't have to sit cross-legged on the floor.

If you have that multi-tasking brain that just won't stifle itself try meditation for even minutes a day allowing thoughts to come and go. The chatter will eventually slow or stop. You also may feel calmer and have less appetite, like a good friend of mine experienced after just two weeks of meditation for the first time at age 56. She is a mover and shaker. Yoga and meditation are not her first choices. If she can do it you can do it!

Brain fog and memory loss may be common in midlife and menopause, but they are not inevitable.

Work in.

63. Eat Fat Keep Muscle

Muscle Protein Synthesis (MPS) is putting the dietary protein you consume to the use of your muscle. Protcin is needed for repairing muscle and preventing losses associated with breakdown from aging and exercise.

The better you are at MPS the more you're spared muscle losses too often associated with "natural" aging. If you can increase your lean muscle, in turn you increase your metabolism. Muscle loss happens easier with age (than muscle gain) and you need to be proactive to offset that, but muscle loss is not inevitable.

One simple way to keep your muscle and fight fat is eat more fat. For MPS it's not just any fat, but Omega 3 fats, that you want according to a study in the American Journal of Clinical Nutrition. Older adults who regularly eat rich sources of Omega-3 fats have increased muscle protein synthesis compared to those who don't. Use food first by eating salmon, tuna or halibut, as long as you're careful about the source. Lamb is also high in Omega 3. Plant sources include flaxseed, hemp hearts and walnuts.

Omega-3 supplements work too, you just want to be sure you're focused on the total EPA and DLA content in the supplement you're taking. Look for at least 1000 mg of those two on the label instead of "other" so you're getting the powerful O-3s dose you want. Read the label to confirm that your Omega 3 supplement is third-party tested for safety and purity.

Omega 3 benefits don't stop at MPS though. In fact they're just getting started. Studies are showing your brain, muscles, and joints all benefit from a boost of Omega 3. They help reduce inflammation too.

64. Pitch the Pink

Yes, pitch pink. The little pink packets, that is. When you think you're reaching for a low-calorie safe alternative to sugar to get or stay slim, you couldn't be more wrong. It's not sweet at all.

Artificial sweetener consumption correlates directly with obesity.

The 200x sweeter chemicals in the little pink or yellow packets or your sugar-free treats are even worse for you than sugar. They can have the same effect on blood sugar and they continue to make you crave more sweets. Give yourself just 11 days to allow your taste buds to change and you'll desire that sweet taste much less. Artificial sweeteners fit under that chemical umbrella that confuses your body. A confused body will slow your metabolism.

Some food for thought from the study that will get your attention:

Diet sodas raised risk of diabetes more than sugar-sweetened sodas.

Women who drank one 12-ounce diet soda had 33 percent increased risk of type 2 diabetes and women who drank one 20 ounce soda had a 66 percent risk.

Women who drank diet sodas drank twice as much as those who drank sugar-sweetened sodas.

If you are trying to justify your own diet soda (or sugar free food) consumption because you're normal weight, consider this next finding.

Artificial sweeteners increased diabetes independent of body weight.

They trick your metabolism into thinking sugar is on its way. This causes your body to pump out insulin, the fat storage hormone, which increases your belly fat.

With diet soda alone, there was a 200% increased risk of obesity in diet soda drinkers.

Then they slow your metabolism down. All the while you're hungrier and you crave even more sugar and starchy carbs like bread and pasta, cookies and cake.

65. Do the Big 3

There are simple rules that will get and keep you slimmer, trimmer, and stronger longer:

- Make 10 minutes.
- Do the biggest needle movers first.
- Do it twice a week.

If you have more than 10 minutes, even better. That first 10 minutes should look very similar no matter if you have 10 minutes, 30 or 60. (Though, really, who has 60 minutes to push weights around any more? The reality is you just don't need it even if you have that kind of time.)

Whether your goals are weight loss, bone density, more energy, or strength the same three exercises matter more. A push, a pull, and a leg exercise make up the big 3 that are your highest priority.

Push: Chest Press, Push Up

Pull: Bent Over Row, Lat Pull Down, Pull Up

Leg: Squat, Leg Press, Lunge (or if your knees say no, hip bridge & ham curl on a ball)

Get in the habit of always making these movers and shakers (or muscles that keep you moving and prevent your parts from shaking and jiggling) your top priority. You can always cut a workout short with confidence you have been consistent in targeting your bones or boosting metabolism.

If you miss some of those small muscle exercises like bicep curls or triceps kickbacks, never fear. Those exercises are frosting but doing them alone will not give you the tone you want in those arms! Gasp?

Truth. You have to stimulate major muscles to get some tone and definition!

The major muscles you use in the big three will to open the door to killer arms by increasing your fat burn all over. You're also not completely neglecting those arm muscles when you use the major muscles either. They're playing back up and still being used.

A recent study* shows that hormone levels are boosted optimally far more with full body workouts than with a "split" routine. That is, if you're doing one or two muscle groups a day to save time, rethink. Unless you're heading to a stage for bodybuilding competition, your midlife metabolism boost is best with a full body workout.

*I want to disclose that this study was not done on midlife women but was clear about the hormonal response that is the significant difference in change. With isolation of body part exercises there was less hormone benefit. Optimal hormone change is necessary to lose the fat and keep the lean.

You can do a full body routine even on busy days in less than 10 minutes. Consistency is your best friend. When time expands, then yes, a more inclusive weight training routine is beneficial. Just keep in mind it's never been about time! It's about the quality of exercise you do. An hour of ho-hum random exercise is far less effective than a high quality focused routine that only takes minutes.

The book bonuses include a weight workout so you can experience the big 3 as top priority with me.

http://bit.ly/2hVs5ep

66. Be Basic But Never Boring

Do you have a black dress in your closet? The little black dress isn't going out of style. Neither is your best exercise plan.

You might think doing squats and lunges would get old after 34 years. When you see and feel results though, you don't fix it if it's not broken! That's what I've been doing.

Cardio alone, as much as we love to rave about interval training, sprint training compared to moderate intensity exercise for longer) ...alone does not significantly boost fat loss. You MUST do strength training. As a woman over 50 who is more easily losing muscle mass than keeping or gaining it, flip a little cardio time into strength for the best body you can have right now and for your future.

Trust me, I've done all the rest in terms of resistance training and cardio options too. I've certified in Pilates (reformer and mat), Yoga, and kickboxing. I've coached triathletes, designed strength and conditioning programs for athletes in golf, volleyball, basketball, gymnastics and I'm probably forgetting a few. I taught high and low impact aerobics, step, and slide, and boot camps featuring tire flipping and battle ropes. After it's all right there waiting for me if I want to use it, I go back to the best investment of my time every time. If I have 10 minutes three times a week I am not going to use my Pilates reformer to boost my metabolism. I am not going to hang my TRX suspension trainer and push, pull, and squat with that. Why?

If you were using Siri to get somewhere wouldn't you want the fastest route? Variety for variety's sake can be a big waste of time that too many women don't have time for today. If you don't use your time doing the thing that will be the most direct path to your goal, you'll lose interest, convince yourself it doesn't work, and you'll give up before you experience results.

Don't get confused. I am all for loving the exercise you do. It's also important that your exercise match your goals. By the time too many women reach me, the mismatch has been part of the problem.

We all need strength training to stay strong, build strong bones, and balance in order to play bigger at those activities we love. A short 20-30 minutes a week (that's all!!) may be all that you need to dedicate to strength training featuring squats and lunges (or a substitute if you're one of my joint girls crying "no!" my joints won't do that!), chest press, and rows.

So you've got this very basic list of exercises to do and you want variety. Here's how to make squats, lunges, chest press, and pulls a little more entertaining and engaging. Use one or more of them to keep things interesting.

- Change the order or sequence of exercises
- Do exercise unilaterally (Perform one arm/one leg at a time)
- Change the tempo (this gives you infinite options: lift/hold/lower/hold)
- Add power (you'll also increase testosterone and increase energy expenditure and bone benefits)
- Change the rest period between exercises
- Change the rest period between sets
- Mix up bilateral (both limbs), unilateral (one limb), and alternating limbs during the same set of exercise

- Use machines at the gym instead of free weights occasionally*
- Try body weight exercises occasionally* *

*I say occasionally because if you choose to exercise at home, you may have just an occasional reason to use a hotel gym or visit with a friend. Don't be afraid to try something new.

**Body weight exercises are a nice challenge but can be limiting as far as ability to reach fatigue in a way that supports bone density or is enough to boost metabolism. Body weight exercises often put more stress on shoulders, and elbows than you want if you've got an existing "niggle." Pulling exercises are also a challenge unless you've got a pull up bar or suspension tool so limit these last two options. They are a great test to your ability to lift your own weight!

67. Take Recovery Seriously

When you don't exercise is just as important as when you do.

Consider that you could exercise 1, 2, or 3 days a week. It's not just the number of workouts. It's the number of days between your workouts that allow you to recover and rebuild before the next one.

For instance, comparing a Monday, Wednesday, Friday workout schedule with a Tuesday Thursday workout schedule only tells you the difference between 2 days a week or 3. There might be a slight difference in the recovery between Friday to Monday vs. Thursday and Tuesday. That could influence the training effect.

What many studies show is very little difference in frequency two days vs. three days of exercise influence on adults over 50. Early studies showed 75% results from twice weekly training.

The widening gap between optimal workouts for younger and older adults really is not about frequency at all. It's about recovery.

There is growing evidence that too little recovery time between workouts prevents full repair of muscles. Even if you did just fine with it a decade ago, you may be more fit now with less frequent exercise.

In fact, when rest and recovery were increased (and protein boosted post exercise: see flip #22) older adults had the ability to work as hard as younger adults and get very similar results.

You may need to abandon traditional exercise class schedules that don't allow for individual recovery needs. If you were doing Monday and Thursday weight training, flip to Monday and Thursday and you may see better results even compared to three weight-training days a week.

Here's the flipping point: You need to earn the rest. Make the exercise significant enough to warrant recovery between exercise sessions.

68. Plan Total Stress Load

It all counts. The good stress and the bad stress all add up. Exercise is stress. Dieting is stress. Life events are stress. Weddings, funerals, and births are all stressors. While we have a heartbeat and meaningful life we won't escape the stress condition. We can plan better to roll with the ups and downs.

When you're falling apart at the seams, shorten your workout or reduce the intensity of the workout.

Do exercise, but don't over do exercise.

While about 80% of people drop exercise all together or reduce it significantly under stress, about 20% turn to exercise to negate the effects of stress. You, ideally, want to be in the middle.

The right movement can reduce your stress level by raising your vibrational energy. Stress, frustration, and depression have low energy vibrations. Good vibrations come from happiness, gratitude and love. So if you love the little movement break you do, you will cope better when you come back to reality.

You just want to make a few considerations.

Your recovery from exercise or tolerance to exercise may change when you're under stress. Your body deals with the all the stress from all sources all the time. When you sense high levels of this "allostatic" stress load consistent but shorter sessions or an extra recovery day between workouts can help. Ditch your scheduled cardio or weights and opt for a walk or yoga instead.

Remember, if you're worried about weight gain or staying on track for loss, it's not about the calories. If you decrease cortisol you will decrease fat storage and help yourself start the fat burning again.

Some signs of stress are obvious: fatigue, headaches, and inability to sleep. Other signs of stress might fly under your radar: more frequent illness and lingering soreness when it's time for your next workout.

It's good to have goals and a plan to reach them. Don't ignore the additional workout that life itself can be and adjust accordingly.

Flipping Point: Avoid the see-how-I-feel workout. Plan your workout along with your meetings and to-do list. Then stick to it. Don't skip it and don't do "extra" because you feel good.

69. Crave the Root Cause

Avoid reading symptoms as your problem. In this case dig deep for information about what you're craving.

Craving salt or sweet? Don't ask, what do I want for a snack, ask why do I have the craving?

It's usually an insufficient amount of micronutrients and or macronutrients.

Dieting typically reduces intake to the point where you can easily become deficient in some key elements. Women who crave chocolate (hello world) may have magnesium deficiency. Given magnesium deficiency is common among women and one of the most often recommended supplements by doctors specializing in women's midlife health it's safe to say, there's a link.

Popcorn is another common food craving for women. Hormone fluctuations, particularly stress hormone fluctuations, are potentially responsible. What do you do instead? You may need B and C vitamins. You also may need meditation, breathing exercises, or a good sweat session! Deal with the stress or emotions as opposed to eat and cause another problem with food.

Fast Flip: Popcorn is not the healthy food you may have been convinced it is. It's full of lectins, potentially fungi, and most corn is genetically modified. It causes inflammation and blood sugar spikes. If you're trading a healthy meal for a bowl of popcorn, you're also trading on your health.

Plan and eat meals with all the good stuff and take supplements to round out your nutrition needs. Few of us can or should eat the over 20,000 calories a day it would take to get all the micronutrients we need. When you're giving your body the food and nutrients it needs and getting pleasure out of enjoying the taste of fresh deliciously prepared food, physiological cravings usually disappear.

Handle your stress and the psychological cravings may also subside. Are you really hungry? Have you just maxed out your willpower for the day and ignored your own needs while tending to everyone else? You're bound to come crashing down if that's true.

I deserve this. It's been a long day.

Who doesn't have the occasional day like that? You're going to start tomorrow feeling lousy if you give into it. There's a good chance you repeat the pattern. You vow to be "good" all day. Then your body and mind naturally make you want exactly what you've avoided.

Do yourself a favor and remove the food from your environment that you'll go to when you have one. For some of my clients it's chocolate chips, for others popcorn. You know you're trigger. For me it's bean chips. I cannot bring them home. They are like crack. Know that if you bring it into your house you intend to eat it. (Others in the household aside. Do ask them to put it where you can't see it.)

Is a snack a bad thing? Not necessarily. Check and recheck your meal content before you decide. Check and recheck your stress and emotions, too. Hormone balance is best when you allow your body to be hungry and recognize fullness. If your busy life made you ignore your signals for too long, they may need a reboot.

70. Reach Fatigue

I'm not very interested in the effect of the menstrual cycle of menopause on exercise. What I am very interested in is the effect of exercise on the menstrual cycle and menopause.

Every woman has a different experience. Even among all of the flipping 50 women from 50-99 we are a diverse group. You want to keep that in mind.

That said, my personal preference is going to leak through if I don't just tell you, I would advise a women lift as heavy as she safely can. That's going to be determined on a joint-by-joint basis. You may have a shoulder or knee issue for instance that reduces what you can do with that joint.

Realistically though heavy weights (even once you progress safely to them) are daunting or risky for some of us. In 2016 there was a study performed on fit young men, yes, note taken. In this case however, it may be relevant to you and I. The study determined that the load of weight lifted didn't change the results of either hypertrophy (gaining muscle fibers) or strength. Both lightweight and heavy weight increased both, as long as one condition was true.

You must reach fatigue.

The overload to the muscles has to be significant enough that you reach the last repetition you can lift, or lift well without risking poor form. That means that yes you can pick up either the 10 lb. weight or the 30 lb. weight as long as you reach fatigue.

No one can tell you how many repetitions that will take. I would recommend no more than 28-30 however. That's a top range for a weight that is most beneficial for gait and power for performance.

This is only true of muscle. For bone benefits you'll want to use a weight heavy enough to reach fatigue in 10 or fewer repetitions, if possible. Your joint-by-joint ability always decides.

Which hormones win? Testosterone and Growth Hormone (GH) that support your lean look and fat loss. If you keep this session short, cortisol also benefits.

Flipping Point: Don't just stop when you reach a certain number of repetitions if you have not reached fatigue.

71. Go DIM

It's no secret you need to eat your veggies. This is one example where that's true but amplifying the goodness in veggies is even better.

Diindolylmethane (DIM) reduces risk of cancers in women due to certain estrogen activity. DIM comes from a bioactive compound derived from cruciferous vegetables. It would take about 4-6 pounds of broccoli and cabbage to have 100-200 mg of DIM. It supports healthy estrogen metabolism by offering a boost if estrogen isn't being metabolized properly because of a toxic liver or poor methylation. DIM helps convert stronger estrogens, which can increase risk for cancer, into protective estrogens.

That's a superpower you want in your life.

It's also a good message about the power of food. Eat more of the right foods and your food truly can be medicine. I'm not suggesting that you shoot for 6 pounds of broccoli today. I am suggesting that you realize every food you put into your body has the potential to make you sicker or healthier.

72. Do It Your Whey

If you tolerate it dairy, use whey protein pre and post exercise not only for your muscle protein synthesis. Whey helps boost glutathione production by up to 64% and helps stabilize blood sugar (taken pre or post exercise).

At other times of day whey is not necessarily your ideal protein shake mix. Whey's easy absorption and digestibility make it ideal pre and post exercise that helps you avoid stomach upset. If you're not exercising and your muscles don't need the fuel whey may spike blood glucose.

That spike can result in insulin that halts fat metabolism and encourages energy story in fat. Try another protein source you tolerate well if you're using protein shakes for snacks or as a convenient meal at times of day when you're not exercising.

The choices can be overwhelming. You could choose between egg, hemp, pea, brown rice, beef, and more. Then there's collagen protein vs. those that offer complete essential amino acids (EAA). Collagen by the way is excellent for connective tissue, gut, and skin but you'll need a protein choice or choices with all the EAA for the muscle sparing benefits you want with a protein shake.

Eliminate options that contain ingredients that you could easily be sensitive to or that could make you fat, or keep you fat. You'll be left with what every woman wants: fewer but better choices. See the next flip for more on ingredients. If you're using one every day as I do, make sure it's serving your flip!

Flipping Point: Test your tolerance to dairy before you buy that big tub or whey. Pause your use of it if you have one. Remove all dairy from your diet for one to three weeks. Then reintroduce it and you may be surprised what you find. Need support? Flipping 50's 28-Day Kickstart walks you through this.

I use a whey smoothie for a pre or post exercise boost to help retain muscle, especially post an intense workout. I tolerate limited amounts of dairy. I use it on a rotation basis and only after challenging sessions to avoid it becoming a food sensitivity for me.

Get the scoop on the right type and timing for protein shakes for your flip.

http://bit.ly/2xsoQCn

73. Read the Label

Protein shakes are a convenient way to get adequate amounts of protein in your diet. I have had a protein smoothie every day for over 20 years. I began using it after every run when I did my first marathon in 1997. Since then I have a breakfast smoothie as a convenient way to pack in more nutrition than I would ever put on a plate.

If you're not carefully selecting your protein shake, however that habit can actually backfire on you. I made that mistake before I knew what I know now. I was using powders containing ingredients I never touch today.

It's one of the reasons after 30 years of saying I would never sell supplements I decided creating a clean product was the responsible thing to do. Women I was working with would realize they needed protein, but not know the difference between good options and bad. Can you imagine using a shake to get lean and spare muscle loss that has ingredients that actually makes you fat?

If you're buying from the health food section at the grocery store, or even a known health food chain, don't blindly assume that they are all equally good. There's much more to consider than the grams of protein or grams of sugar in a protein shake.

Artificial sweeteners, sugar, artificial flavors, soy, chemicals, and gums, can all make a protein shake backfire on you. Heavy metals and arsenic have been found in 50% of randomly tested protein powders. Some of the most popular brands of protein shakes are full of the ingredients above. Imagine you're sitting down to a serving of chicken or fish (vegans bear with me). Would you want it to have been pumped full of maltodextrin, sucralose, and soy or artificial flavors?

Fast Flip: If you have a protein shake right now, go read the label and see if it passes the "clean" test.

- The fewer ingredients the better
- All ingredients pronounceable
- The less sugar the better (5 grams or less)
- Void of chemicals (look up ingredients you don't recognize)
- No artificial anything
- Beware of "natural" ingredients especially tucked in a long list (this can be used to describe sugar)

Would you give it to your children?

Fast Flip: You may be wondering about my mention of soy on the hit list. Soy is an obesogen (causing obesity), an estrogenic (interrupting estrogen function), and a goitrogenic. There's evidence it increases fat storage and decreases fat burning as well as disrupts endocrine (hormone) and thyroid function. For many of my clients, even living in Japan eating high quality soy, eliminating soy reduced hot flashes and night sweats. That made it possible to sleep.

I would be remiss not to tell you there is a flip side to the soy story and my friend, Dr. Lindsey Berkson, is a leading hormone authority believes in the benefit of soy. I've included her website in the resources. Ultimately, the best thing you can do is test. Don't guess.

74. Get Busy

When it comes to equality of the sexes, where sex benefits are concerned, you win. Women win. You have more feel good hormones and you have more (than men) reduced risk of cardiovascular disease.

Before I go on may I just point out how proud of that first sentence I am? Puns intended all the way through. If discussions of sex disturb you, skip this flip. Disclaimer: it's not G rated.

If you're not getting any you may want to start. Your hormone balance depends on it. Here's the short list of hormones that will be better for it if you fool around regularly.

Growth hormone increases. That's more muscle for you.

Estrogen production increases. That's a number of things including better skin, less belly fat and bone loss.

Testosterone increases. More confidence and less muscle loss.

Oxytocin (the cuddle hormone) increases. You bond.

Endorphins increase. You feel good.

Serotonin increases. You feel even better.

Cortisol is reduced lowering your perceived stress level.

These hormone benefits combined mean you'll be in a better mood, get more regular periods if you're still having them, you'll feel closer to your partner and experience less stress. Your skin may clear, and in fact glow, and you can get better results from that workout and those nutritious foods you're consuming.

Can you make all this happen yourself? Not to the same extent as if you're with a partner.

How much is enough? Enjoy sex three times a week in your 50's and you may give up Botox injections. Research suggests the 50-something that makes love with this frequency looks up to 10 years younger.

You might also fix that pesky menopause acne thanks to a response that reduces inflammation. Bonus!

Are you competitive? Frequency of sex is apparently declining for so many reasons: stress, texting instead of talking, and exposure to toxins to name a few. Collectively we're all having sex less than we did a decade ago. The older you are though the worse it gets. A 20-something adult has sex 80 times a year and by the time she's 80 it's down to 20 times a year.

Is it the get in shape mojo you need? It could be. More sexually active adults have a better body or at least body image. Which happens first? Are you motivated to take better care of yourself to increase pleasure or do you get a better body from sex?

You know what I say. Test. Don't guess.

Part III

Hot, Not Hurt or Bothered Flips

75. Brand Your Exercise

At least 80% of women would benefit from a custom program that includes attention to their weak links, and a hormone-exercise connection program based on their personal signs and symptoms. Don't misconstrue that to think you may be in the 20% that doesn't need a custom exercise plan. That 20% already has a custom program!

Even in a woman's-only exercise program, one designed for women over 50, each individual in the program has unique needs. You require a different set of work-to-recovery intervals, a different load of weight training based on your body type, or your goals. Your sequence or tempo may need a tweak.

Have you started an exercise class or boot camp with a friend or spouse? Did you notice one of you got results faster than the other? While you were attending the same sessions, doing the same exercises you got different results? Then you know the truth about a one-size-fits-all exercise plan.

Your exercise needs are as unique as your thumbprint. No longer do we believe a room full of people, can do the same exercise routine and expect to get the same results.

I'm often asked, what's the best exercise? I'm _____. (Insert age)

Truth is that it has very little to do with age and everything to do with ability. Your health status, history, current exercise, time demands, stressors, and your goals.

Even if the question is, what's the best exercise to lose weight? I'm ___.

The missing piece is "for me right now."

If you're surrounded by women in a group exercise program with one instructor calling out the same instruction to everyone in the room, ask yourself if you have the same life experience, health history, fitness level, and goals and conditions as everyone else.

Recovery time is especially unique to each of us. You may require slightly more recovery time both between sessions and between sets & repetitions than your younger self, or than others in your group. If you're using an imposed class schedule, cadence or music, you're less likely to have these options.

Listen to your body. Fatigued? Sore? Do you feel weaker at subsequent workouts than you should be? If so, try another day of rest (instead of another day of exercise) and you may be pleasantly surprised that your fitness improves.

Flipping Point: Design your exercise to be as unique as you.

76. Get the Right High

Talking about the runner's high may give you flashbacks to the 70's and 80's when the running movement was first making waves. The endorphin rush from exercise still alive and well but comes in different doses related to the intensity of your exercise. A study in Neuropsychopharmacology found the release of feel good hormones is uniquely tied to intensity of exercise, and perhaps to your fitness status.

Moderate and high intensity exercise produces the most feel good opioid release. Extremely high exercise intensities also produce negative emotions. So you've got to be cautious.

At the highest exercise intensities the release of endorphins may happen to overcome negative feelings and discomfort required to get through the work. Your body works to protect you in every way! Little shots of high intensity exercise (think High Intensity Interval Training or HIIT) as opposed to trying to sustain long bouts may help you over come this. If you're of average weight and moderately fit you may enjoy a bigger mental boost from high intensity exercise.

On the other hand, if you're overweight or obese weight, self-selecting your exercise intensity shows up as important. Don't let a trainer or "zone training" suggest to you where you need to be to burn the most fat. You've got to have a habit in the first place to have it do any good. Moderate training intensities might encourage more overall pleasure associated with exercise and help you keep the habit.

Either way, pleasure and euphoria are words you want to associate exercise with!

Fast Flip: Take two minutes and plan your exercise this week. If endorphins can make you "high" they can also be addictive. Seeking a quick HIIT too often is hard on muscles and encourages breakdown. Put one HIIT on the calendar if it's new for you. Test twice weekly if you've adapted, as long as there are recovery days between them. More is not always better.

If your inner voice is telling you to pull up your big girl panties and do more, don't. Even elite athletes don't do more than one or two HIIT sessions a week. They're better for it.

Injury rates go up faster than fitness at a certain point. Your certain point is unique to you. Your just right is another Flipping 50 babe's too much. Take rest days between those intense workouts. A lot of good flips still happen at lower intensity movement.

77. Opportunity Knocks: Answer

If you exercise regularly, you have a better opportunity to spare muscle losses. All it takes is strategically increasing your protein intake after exercise. A study in Medicine & Science in Sports & Exercise showed adults 65-80 experienced increased muscle protein synthesis (MPS) immediately after exercise.

That means your ability to use protein to your advantage is increased for about 24-30 hours and possibly as long as 48-72 hours after exercise. You have a one-two punch to help you not only prevent muscle losses, but potentially to gain lean muscle if you need it. This gives you an edge over inactive adults your same age that even if they increase their protein intake, won't be able to use it as well.

If you exercise most days of the week, provided it's of adequate intensity, (moderate to vigorous) you're almost always in an "acute" post-exercise anabolic state. That allows you to build muscles up and prevents them from breaking down. All you need to do is stay conscious of including high quality protein at each meal and snack to help. It can be a delicious problem.

Your body will use protein in these post exercise windows more optimally than on your rest days. So reach for the nut butter, the turkey, or my personal favorite, a smoothie and boost your lean bottom line.

Here's my favorite again.

Chocolate Mint Smoothie

Chocolate Paleo Power or Plant Power Protein Shake

½ frozen banana
¼ avocado
handful of spinach
1 T raw cacao powder
1 tsp Mint Greens
1 tsp Fiber Boost
Small amounts of unsweetened almond, cashew, or coconut milk to thickness
ice

Make it thin and drink it or thick and top it:

- Cacao nibs
- Sliced almonds
- Raw coconut

My clean ingredients:

http://bit.ly/2fX5pWR

78. Question Everything

Your hormones, body composition, metabolism and socialization are all different from a male. Yet only 39% of all sport and exercise studies are done on women.

According to a study of 1382 sports and exercise medicine articles involving 6,076,580 participants in The European Journal of Sport Science you're not represented.

Think about the implications of this. Most textbooks and certification courses for courses your personal trainer and fitness instructor takes are based on research done on men, most of them fit young men. That means that most programs are designed for men even if they're marketed with an image of a woman or made a women's-only class.

We need to re-evaluate the reasons we're exercising in the way we are and whether it was based on some of the emerging research that is based on midlife women or not.

Be a critical thinker when news about a study catches your attention. It may or may not be relevant. Were the subjects like you?

Ask:

Were the subjects female?

Were the subjects my age?

Were the subjects my fitness status?

Was this a large pool of subjects?

A few short years ago a study proved that exercise in a fasted state (before breakfast) burned more fat than the same exercise done later in the day after a meal. The news went out that exercising fasted was the best fat burner.

Never mind that the study was done on fit young men who were being fed an extremely high calorie, 50% fat diet. So would that be applicable to you if you were watching your calories and eating moderate or low amounts of fat? You have to wonder.

We do by nature tend to follow leaders who are going in the direction we already wanted to go in. When we blindly follow studies and research that fit the way we believed, it may just be that we wanted to be right. We like to be right.

Read. Listen. Question it. Then test it.

79. Ask the right question

If the questions you're asking yourself are negative, "Why can't I get motivated?" or you're telling yourself "I just have no discipline," ask "Do I want that to be true?"

If the answer is no, change the question. Ask, "What do I need to help me be more accountable?" or "what's something I can do I love and can look forward to?" If your energy level keeps you from doing more ask, "what do I need to know to have more energy?"

Change is stressful. Under stress you can be limited in your ability to problem solve. But positive affirmations, even in the form of questions can counter the negative affects of stress.

As an online fitness professional many customers who reach out to our support staff tend to default to, "What I am doing wrong?" As many as 9/10 women in fact who reach out because they can't find what they want or can't apply a coupon code, will default to assuming it's them!

Just 1 out of 10 will imply it's our site not working. That offers some insight into how we might be thinking about anything the rest of the day. When your fitness and personal health goals aren't going right, do you assume it's your own lack of willpower or discipline?

You don't think first that it might be the program or the diet but you blame you? Not helpful.

By flipping the negative reel playing inside your head over and over you stop the negative stream so you can replace it with a more positive message.

Try a rubber band around the wrist. Snap it when you realize you've sent yourself a negative memo.

80. Check Leucine

You're losing muscle easier than you're gaining it. Protein is necessary to maintain and build muscle. Essential Amino Acids (EAA) in proteins specifically stimulate muscle protein synthesis. EAAs then become your new best friend.

Leucine, specifically is one of the most important EAAs. It's most prevalent in whey protein shakes. Eggs are also an excellent source. Know what you tolerate by testing in order to seek the best sources for you personally. Other animal sources also have leucine in fairly high amounts. Plant-based protein sources high in leucine are harder to find.

Results of a study can show just how important leucine is to your fat-to-lean ratio. Even when a lower than optimal dose (15 g) of essential amino acids were ingested as long as leucine levels were high (2.8 g) protein synthesis remained high. When leucine levels dropped to 1.7 g protein synthesis also dropped. Prior studies indicate 2.3 g of leucine per serving for beneficial muscle protein synthesis.

Fast Flip: If you're using a protein shake mix, check the label or connect with the manufacturer and ask about the amount of leucine per serving. Even I don't include that directly on my label but have the information ready for those who ask. Your Whey is highest, Paleo Power (beef) protein is next, and Plant Power (pea) has the lowest.

Supplementing with EAA may be appropriate for you if:

- Your training is exercise significant

You have lost a lot of muscle tissue and have a hard time gaining it back

You have anxiety

Check with your physician before you supplement with EAA. High protein for those with existing kidney conditions is not advised.

81. Power Up

Lift heavy things fast. Speed and strength together make power. If that sounds like an injury waiting to happen, it's not. You're going to lift very quickly and still lower under control. You're never swinging or allowing momentum to take over.

Power engages your fast twitch muscle fibers. Those are the ones responsible for dashing upstairs, catching a falling child, or preventing yourself from falling on a little patch of ice or water on the floor. They help you pull open a heavy door, or catch one that's been caught by a strong wind.

Falls in older adulthood are preventable with a higher level of power. It starts now. Not motivated by something that might help you in 20 years? Then consider this. Have you ever seen a fat sprinter? That's power. Are you with me again?

Lifting heavy weight with power provides you with the most benefits in all areas: power, strength, and endurance. Lifting slow on the other hand only provides you with strength. For you, busy hot babe, spending your weight training time using power will get you more results in less time.

What is heavy? It's a weight that you can't lift more than about 10 times. That's the equivalent of 80% of a 1 Repetition Maximum (1-RM). You'd never want to actually do a 1-RM: it's not safe. It's also not necessary.

Someone already did the heavy lifting for you in studies that found 10 repetitions correspond with 80% of a 1-RM. That number has significance not just for helping boost lean muscle and burn fat, but using power with a heavy weight also provides the best bone density benefits.

Power also increases energy expenditure. You get stronger, you get less likely to fall, and you get smaller.

How do you get there?

Start with a lightweight you can lift 15-20 times.

Do exercises slow and controlled. Lift 1-2 counts and lower 3-4 counts.

Progress to a weight you can lift 12-15 times.

Progress to a weight you can lift 10 or fewer times.

(Progress every two weeks after doing twice per week sessions.)

Then you begin to add power by lifting quickly, and continuing to lower slowly so you keep the weight under your control.

If you've been lifting weights and have a foundation of strength, try it today and see if you feel the difference. You can do this with machines, free weights, or cables.

82. Don't Go Nuts

Love nuts? If you get carried away and find yourself eating them in the morning and afternoon that snack habit may be tied to your aching knees.

The high Omega 6 to Omega 3 ratio in nuts may be increasing your inflammation.

Once we learned nuts were healthy, many of us overdid them. They have high levels of Omega 6 fats. Munching on nuts occasionally is fine. If you're doing it daily, and enjoying nut butter, and maybe doing nuts and or seeds in the morning and the afternoon, that healthy habit could backfire. Omega 6 fats turn on the inflammation faucet Omega 3 fats turn it off.

Most food sources of Omega 3 also contain a higher amount of Omega 6. That's the case with nuts. It's tricky. Since reducing internal inflammation is an important first step to better health and optimal weight, assess your intake of nuts and seeds. Reduce that. Increase your Omega 3 supplement to help offset this ratio.

Look for "third party tested" on your fish oil label. Some reports of rancid fish oils mean you could be increasing your inflammation instead of decreasing it if you don't choose carefully.

I find with a lot of physical training stress or joint aches and pains an increased amount of Omega 3s improves healing and reduces discomfort.

If you're at risk for disease or have breast cancer, or rheumatoid arthritis there are ratios of Omega 6/Omega 3 defined as more optimal and those that increase risk.

For example a study reported a 4:1 ratio of omega 6: omega 3 reduced mortality from cardiovascular disease by 70%. In breast cancer the ratio of 2.5:1 reduced risk and for rheumatoid arthritis 2-3:1 suppressed inflammation. On average most adults consume ratios closer to 20:1.

Be proactive with regard to awareness of your intake of Omega 6 fats and offset it with Omega 3 supplementation as needed.

83. Dance

Ditch your long endurance love affair and have a short intense fling. Testosterone levels tank with long endurance activity while cortisol increases to a detrimental level. Unless you have a reason – a passion, you're a paid athlete – and you've progressed slowly to longer sessions and love the body you're living in, the brain function, mood, and sleep you're getting - try shorter workouts with greater intensity the majority of the time you exercise.

Even if you do have a long endurance event, try shorter interval sessions. I put this new training to the test this fall. In fact, as I write this I'm less than two months from an Ironman distance triathlon. I wanted to test the impact of training long on my hormones after having balanced them doing short intense sessions 80% of the time for the past 3 years.

Instead of traditional longer training sessions I'm breaking them up. My run today was two miles in the morning, two at noon, and two in the evening. It was a shorter total distance (I cut a 9 mile run) and less draining on the hormone tank this way. I'll post results in a second edition or you can find it on the blog at Flippingfifty.com.

Beware of that tendency to do too much of a good thing. By short intense fling I'm referring to the duration of each high intensity interval training (HIIT) workout. Keep it short. You also don't want to do this every day. One or two times a week a high intensity session is good, but more is not better. If you do add a third session (once your body has adapted) look for signs that you're slipping backwards: soreness, fatigue, more aches and pains. If you don't feel fully recovered starting your next workout, wait.

A long exercise session that's planned and is preceded by proper progression can be a good hormone balancer too. When you begin to go longer than 75 minutes cortisol levels tend to rise. Watch for signs and symptoms you don't recover well. Those include you're more tired but may not be able to sleep or more hungry instead of invigorated.

When cortisol is elevated hormones that provide optimal lean muscle and less fat, (testosterone, growth hormone, and insulin) are depressed. You want to exercise to optimally employ them all at the right levels: enough but not too much. Your job is to dance with intensity so well that you you don't elevate cortisol too much and you elevate testosterone, growth hormone, and insulin enough.

You have a sweet spot unique to you. Don't let me, or anyone else, tell you exactly what you should do unless we're working together in a coaching relationship. You'll need to test yourself and listen to signs and symptoms that you need to two-step a little differently.

Got the book bonuses? You'll get the Interval Training 101 inside!

http://bit.ly/2hVs5ep

84. Prime Yourself

Karen recruited me as her personal trainer because she was exercising without seeing any results. When she showed me what she'd been doing it became crystal clear why she wasn't losing weight or tone, her goals, from her weight training. It wasn't the exercises. It wasn't the sequence.

It was the weight.

Karen had read and heard in classes that she needed to do 15 repetitions. She did two or three sets of each of the exercises and just stopped when she got to 15. She wasn't at fatigue. She wasn't even close.

I asked her how she was feeling at the end of every set.

"Could you do five more?"

"Yes."

She did them.

"Could you do five more?"

"Yes."

She did them too.

At that very first session I asked her to do a few more if she felt she could. I ended up stopping her at 30! She still wasn't at fatigue.

We built up Karen's confidence and then over a couple weeks got her to a weight where she was doing 10-15 repetitions to fatigue. If she didn't fatigue at that weight by 15 in two consecutive workouts, we had her increase her weight so that she did.

Four weeks later, Karen had lost 4 inches overall and she was wearing pants from the back of the closet.

Karen is not alone!

Women self-select weights that are below the threshold of recommendations even for good health: way below! Performing the recommendations for good health is the bare minimum to prevent disease and remain independent in daily activities of living.

We need to lift at least 60% of a 1-Repetition Maximum (or the equivalent of being able to lift 25-30 times). What older women tend to choose is between 33-51% for common exercises.

Here's the kicker: When women are blindfolded they easily lift much more weight than they say they can. What you think, or how you prime yourself, matters. I've caught myself underestimating what I can do. I will habitually go in and lift the weights I'm used to lifting. One day recently there were two extra plates on the leg press, increasing the load SIGNIFICANTLY! I did it, got up and only then did I notice what I'd done. I sat down thinking about how it would feel, and it did. It didn't feel heavier.

If you're lifting so light you can do more than 30 of anything alarms should go off! Using weights that light will fail to give you strength, bone density, and lean muscle that boosts your metabolism.

You don't have time to waste! So it's important that you're starting with a lighter, safe weight and then progressing. If you're able to do more repetitions when you get to the end of a set, it's time to increase the weight.

Fast Flip: Good starting ranges for beginners and then for progressing approximately every two weeks if all is going well follow. If you have a special condition err on the conservative side and check with a Medical Exercise Specialist for support.

Super Light: 25-30 repetitions

Light 15-20 repetitions

Medium 12-15 repetitions

Heavy 10 or fewer repetitions

85. Sleep Sound

If your number one wish in the world is for a good night's sleep, this is for you. It takes sleep to get better results from exercise. The right exercise at the right time can also help your sleep.

Sleep quality improves with exercise. Moderate intensity wins over low-level exercise for improving your sleep quality. In this particular study yoga, for example, didn't result in significant sleep quality change. Part of that may be the heat regulation difference between low intensity and moderate or higher intensity exercise. Exercise that induces sweat and encourages heat dissipation can help avoid night sweats

Are you wondering about your hot yoga or power yoga practice? The research on yoga is all over the place, honestly. In part that's due to the many types of yoga and the variability in delivery, students, teachers and temperature. If you swear by yoga for benefits like stress relief and calming mental chatter, then go for it. Don't ditch other forms of exercise though. If you've not started yoga, focus first on heart pumping exercise that gets you a little breathless and add yoga next.

You may not get more sleep because of exercise but you can increase the quality of your shuteye. Many of my students however do increase the length of their sleep time by as much as two hours compared to pre-program sleep. That may be because they consciously make the decision to go to sleep when they are tired. Instead of trying to tackle more on your "to do" list or giving up your power to a movie, watch what happens when you get the rest your body craves.

Sleep quality and quantity both directly influence hormones that increase lean muscle, decrease fat storage, and reduce cravings. Moderate intensity exercise should be a high priority if you're sleepless too often.

Sleep Yourself Skinny is full of suggestions for how you can get more sleep.

http://bit.ly/2fIdzCv

86. Bone Up

In 2017 a simple truth was revealed about bone health. Since 1995 the dietary focus for better bones had been on calcium and Vitamin D through foods and supplements. The reality is in alignment with everything we know about health and fitness: you can't look at any one thing in isolation any more. You're an integrated being.

The big reveal is this: all diet is crucial for bone health.

It's not only calcium, nor the addition of D, but a diet rich overall in high quality macronutrients (fats, protein, carbohydrates) and micronutrients is required to have optimal bone health.

One study showed due to the increased potassium and manganese daily prune consumption improved bone density. Another study proved increasing intake of vegetables and fruits enhanced the overall micronutrient sufficiency of iron, boron, selenium, and copper, which in turn enhanced bone health.

Support for bone remodeling comes from decreasing oxidative stress on the body overall.

Bone health isn't an isolated job. Building bones is a part of the overall orchestration of the human body. If you focus not on weight loss, fat loss, but instead on optimal function it will result in optimal bones, body weight, and skin, hair, nails and energy.

Strong bones are an important part of maintaining an active lifestyle. Bone losses begin at age 30. Building bone and slowing losses gets more challenging though not impossible with age. A decline in estrogen during menopause accelerates bone loss during that 3-5 year period so it's important to prepare, or to act now to up level your overall nutrition status on behalf of your bones.

87. Power with Plant

Old school thoughts of supplementing with Calcium and Vitamin D to increase Bone Mineral Density are giving way to new and potentially healthier options. Oddly though calcium is known to the public as the end-all bone solution, numerous studies show supplementation has no correlation with increased bone density or reduced risk of fractures. Conversely, calcium supplementation is connected directly to heart disease and other health risk.

Bone spurs and constipation often come up in reference to calcium supplements. The studies are contradictory and inconclusive from my research. There doesn't seem to be a connection with bone spurs and calcium documented but several health practitioners I know have noted patients they see with bone spurs also take calcium.

There's a new kid on the block. Sea algae-based products may have the potential to increase bone density. Whereas in most studies the significance of an intervention is based on a control group that is losing bone to subjects who don't lose bone, a human study published in 2011 involving more than 200 women ages 18-85 increased bone density by more than 2% on average.

To gain bone density at all once you're an adult is unusual. The pre and post measurements were done six months apart.

Along with assessing the BMD outcome the study measured safety of the supplement. There was no evidence of cardiovascular risk or any of diminished results over time. It might be the gift you want that does keep giving. In 2016, results of a 7-year longitudinal trial were published further backing this plant-sourced calcium supplement. The product is AlgaeCal and I have no affiliation.

88. Resist Bone Loss

Depending on your age, stage of peri, menopause, or post menopause you have a unique potential to either build bone or protect it.

Even when bone building becomes less likely post menopause, slowing or preventing losses is a worthy goal.

Improving strength is also a key priority. Balance and posture focused exercises should round out a program for you if you're top priority is bone health or preventing fractures.

I've poured over research since 1996 on bone density. I've read, watched, and listened to doctors, trainers, and women like you share information about bone health.

There are a lot of messages going out, not necessarily in alignment with the primary research. So this is it. From the most recent studies existing the consensus is that high intensity resistive strength training provided maximum benefit.

The benefits of high intensity (or high force) resistance training were directly to bone mineral density (BMD), muscle mass, and resulted in a reduction in fractures.

Secondary to resistance training in importance for low bone density, or osteoporosis, are posture and balance exercises. Those only improved mobility and did not directly support bone or muscle improvement. That said, mobility that supports ease in movement and the ability to right yourself if you lose balance can be extremely important in preventing falls. It is the building of BMD that will help prevent fracture in the event of a fall.

When or if you are diagnosed with osteoporosis fear can follow quickly behind. You may fear a fracture. You may also fear getting hurt from the very exercise that will benefit your bones. You're smart to feel that way. I want to emphasize that not resistance training carries far greater risk than not resistance training. You inevitably will lose more muscle and more bone at a faster rate without it. That will cause weakness and loss of balance and strength. That will cause loss of confidence.

Shall we skip the rest of the doom and gloom? You do have a great deal of power to influence your health from resistance training. It is not only your bones that will benefit but also every aspect of your life including sleep, stress, anxiety levels, energy, stamina and cognitive health.

To put your fear to rest, the study showed performing high force exercises did not increase fractures and were associated with BMD increases.

What is the definition of high force resistance training? Using a weight you can lift in a lower range of repetitions (10 or fewer) to fatigue fits this description. If you currently have osteoporosis and are new to exercise this is not a starting point. It's a place you'll progress to over weeks and potentially months.

It's important to note that low intensity programs provided less pronounced benefits initially and lead to increased fall risk. In a 10-year follow up on subjects who did low intensity programs however, they did show evidence of reduced fractures in one study.

Flipping Point: Every exercise has health benefits. Not every exercise has bone benefits. The most optimal exercise for BMD is high intensity resistance training. If you have limits that deem this unsafe or impractical, do the next best thing.

Do you want more support for bone health?

http://bit.ly/2gryc6M

89. Exercise IBS Caution

Should you exercise on an empty stomach? Should you eat before exercise? If you should eat, what should you eat?

These questions are common. Behind them is often something deeper than whether or not you'll burn the most fat if you do or don't eat. Active women, and women athletes, have a higher prevalence of Irritable Bowel Syndrome (IBS) than men do. Hormones strike again.

The answer to those questions about eating is, it depends. I'll share some information here about the right type of fuel for the right type of activity. I want you to realize though that "you are the boss of you." I think we can both agree on that. You are the expert on what works. If you feel nauseas or heavy if you eat first, even following guidelines on easy-to-digest foods, then wait. On the other hand if you get shaky, or feel weak, or you're distracted due to hunger, having something in your gut will help.

You may be one of the unlucky ones with worse issues. Severe gut pain or sudden diarrhea can strike as they please. Here's my personal story.

I used to never eat before I exercised. I'd have coffee and go. And I often suffered big time. I can remember being in Madrid, Spain, and on the island of Maui in Hawaii barely making it back to our hotel room because I was doubled over with gut pain in the middle of a run. Then there was the time I was running with my husband on a country road in Iowa and I was so sick he had to flag down some random farmer and ask for a ride back to our hotel.

I was adverse about eating before. I felt lighter on empty. Once I began adapting to eating before runs I had fewer and less severe gut issues. Most runners, especially females, have the occasional trouble. It's rare for me now.

Flipping point: Be open to change if what you're doing now isn't really working.

The truth about the best way to fuel for the hot, not bothered babe in you is to match the fuel plan to the activity. High intensity workouts will use some carbohydrate for fuel. So starting with a little carb before can help light the fire that will burn fat on the back end.

I like a hearty (not cardboard) brown rice cake with almond or sun butter, or some toasted sweet potato slices with nut butter and cinnamon.

For longer slower sessions (the hormone balancing kind, not the hour of power you used to do on cardio equipment), eat minimally if you can. If you opt for something have fat and or a fat/protein combination. Your body will burn more fat for fuel if it's empty but you don't want to start out hungry.

I like ¼ to ½ an avocado or some nuts pre-exercise if I'm eating before a long hike or long easy bike ride. Give yourself a little time to digest. Do avoid fiber and roughage for moderate and greater intensity exercise. That's the only time you'll get me to say that!

Test yourself.

90. Enjoy After Burn

This is about the power of exercise to keep boosting your metabolism for hours after you're showered. It's a beautiful thing. You may be reminded of Flip #77 here.

It takes 15 to 48 hours for the body to fully recover after exercise. We exercise physiologists call this Excess Post Exercise Oxygen Consumption, or EPOC. There's such a wide time span because it depends on the intensity and the duration of the exercise.

Why is that important to you? Because your body is burning far more calories (and fat) during this time than it typically does at rest. So if you're sitting on your bum right now reading, and you've exercised earlier today or possibly even yesterday you are in the bonus round still burning more than if today was purely sedentary.

In a review of studies to find whether duration or intensity mattered more, the clear winner is intensity. I repeat, the intensity of an aerobic exercise bout has the greatest impact on EPOC. As intensity increases the magnitude and duration of EPOC increases.

Read all the way to the end of this flip! You may get caught up in the benefit of aerobic training in these early paragraphs. If you're excited about that, you're going to be flipping over the resistance training nail-biter ending.

The study in question examined exercise intensities of 29%, 50%, and 75% exercise done for the same period of time (80 minutes). The 75% intensity resulted in the greatest EPOC magnitude and duration. EPOC lasted 10 hours as opposed to .3 and 3.3 hours, respectively for 29% and 50% activity.

What's 29% feel like? Less than it would take you to go up and downstairs with baskets full of laundry or groceries.

What's 50%? Still very comfortable and a level you can talk in full sentences easily. This is a leisure walk with the (small to medium not-so-peppy) dog.

At 75% you know you're working. In fact, you're a little curious about how long you'll need to do it. You're breathing harder and talking between breaths. Given the choice you'd rather ask questions than talk.

Testing the same energy expenditure during exercise at different intensities the exercise sessions for each intensity would be different durations. Even when that variation was tested so the exact same number of calories were burned at each of three intensities the EPOC was almost double with the higher intensity exercise than at the lower intensity.

Interval training EPOCs compared to continuous exercise were 60% greater.

That doesn't mean don't take those longer walks. For hormone balance they are still important to you. Incorporating high intensity intervals into continuous exercise significantly increase EPOC, though. About half way through a longer walk, do 5-8 short bursts of faster walking or hill repeats (charge up for a minute and walk back down) and then carry on.

Here's where the tide turns back to your miracle makeover. Last but not least, researchers compared three activities:

- Heavy resistance training (3-8 reps, 8 exercises, at 80-90%)
- Circuit training (4 sets, 8 exercises, 15 reps at 50%)
- Aerobic exercise bout

Have you already guessed? Heavy resistance training produced the most EPOC. This study also backs up other proof that longer rest intervals are an important variable.

Rest for 120 seconds vs. 30 seconds between heavy training and circuit training sets to get greater EPOC.

91. Do Less, Better

Exercise for women in menopause is tricky. Short intense bouts of exercise can increase Human Growth Hormone (HGH) and testosterone, and these help you increase lean muscle that boost metabolism. Too much of a good thing however will backfire on you.

Long duration moderate and high intense activity increase cortisol. During menopause your body is much more susceptible to negative impact of cortisol.

Relaxing activities don't burn as many calories but if they reduce cortisol you improve your ability to lose weight and reduce the storage of fat caused by elevated cortisol. So yes, do those interval training sessions. Just don't let yourself think that if 20 minutes is good 40 minutes is better. It's not.

Don't completely discount low-level activity. When a reset is what you need, returning to walking might be exactly what you need. Walking outdoors anywhere is helpful, but in nature is most helpful compared to walking city streets, at reducing cortisol. Substitute your equivalent of walking if need be. Enjoy biking, canoeing, hiking, paddle boarding? Go for it. Head to the park if you're in the city, and definitely take advantage of those country roads if that's where you live.

92. Exercise for Chronic Fatigue

Chronic Fatigue Syndrome goes beyond mild fatigue many women in midlife experience (and some of us are aces at ignoring). CFS includes trouble sleeping, joint aches and muscles aches, sore throat, concentration problems, dizziness, not feeling rested from sleep, unusual headaches, extreme exhaustion. These usually go on for six months or more to define CFS. Adrenal fatigue and chronic fatigue are not the same but there's some overlap. Some level of adrenal fatigue may contribute to CFS.

The exact cause is not known and so, as you'd guess the solution isn't either. All of the suggestions in this book however including changing and testing dietary needs, buffing up your sleep routine, and testing exercise make sense.

Menopause symptoms often mimic chronic fatigue syndrome (CFS). Certainly if you have CFS it may be amplified during menopause. Should you exercise when you're already tired?

Yes, seems to be the answer. Exercise improves general well being and there is no evidence that it will worsen symptoms.

Depression, anxiety, sleep, and pain reports didn't change significantly with exercise program participation. There were overall reductions in fatigue.

The specific type, intensity, and duration, of exercise that helps the most is still unknown. It may be unique to you. The best way to learn about what works for you is:

Start with activity you enjoy. Try a convenient and easy option like walking or using a stationary bike to reduce impact, or turn on music and dancing in your living room.

Start with short duration, low level, moderate frequency and progress alternately in intensity and frequency. Try 10 minutes a couple times a week the first week. Increase to 15 minutes the next. Do it three days the following week, and so on.

Pay attention to your own fatigue, sleep, mood and pain symptoms. Continually assess yourself to find that sweet spot. Be OK with doing just 10 minutes most days a week if that is where you experience benefits without feeling "hung over" from the exercise. Think of it like a dose of any medicine: frequent consistent doses get the best results.

Exercise early in the day to improve or, at least, not disrupt sleep.

A combination of aerobic and weight training exercise have the most potential to influence mood as each offers unique positive effects.

Weight training for instance increases self-esteem, boosts brain function, and enhances posture. Aerobic exercise also increases self-esteem, serves as a distraction from stressors, and boosts mood with the notorious endorphins released during and after exercise.

Even with all the benefits of aerobic and weight training, don't overlook less stimulating and more mindful exercise like yoga for beginning if these feel like too much.

93. Blast Fat Fast?

Chances are you have a strong opinion about Intermittent Fasting (IF) or you are searching for more information about it. I'll give you my honest opinion right from the start so there's no confusion. It's a huge risk where midlife women are concerned. The cons outweigh the pros when I assess physiological and psychological changes that occur during and after fasting.

The biggest drawback is that this flirts with a binge-purge cycle too reminiscent of eating disorders. Starting IF without having a good relationship with food, and a foundation of the right foods for your optimal energy and gut health just sets you up for a fall.

There's no arguing that a hormone helpful in releasing fat (glucagon) is increased after fasting. However, very few studies have been done with midlife women already more susceptible to the negative effects of stress (due to a vast change occurring in a least half a dozen hormones). Studies done on young, healthy men can't be directly applied to women in their 40s-60s.

You're messaging your body all the time. You're either telling it to burn more calories when you eat more, or to burn less when you eat less or not at all. You're telling your body to burn more calories when you exercise. Confused with two conflicting messages, your metabolism tends to slow. Your body gets more efficient operating on less. It will hold onto fat and fat storage becomes a priority as your body tries to protect you from whatever may have limited your food supply, even if it's your choice.

All that said. I am compelled to be fair and share with you the other side of the research. Some of my respected colleagues swear by IF for themselves. Your job is to be a critical thinker about where you are and what's true of your relationship with food before you decide. A study in the Journal of Midlife Health states the biggest issue with IF lies in the lack of clinical studies due to ethics. In other words, because there is risk in having subjects fast for extended periods of time, few if any studies exist on midlife women that can shed light on immediate or long-term effects.

This is the science. Studies of IF (e.g., 60% energy restriction on 2 days per week or every other day), Part time Fasting (e.g., a 5-day diet providing 750-1100kcal) and time-restricted feeding (TRF; limiting the daily period of food intake to 8h or less) in normal and overweight human subjects have demonstrated efficacy for weight loss and improvements in multiple health indicators including insulin resistance and reductions in risk factors for cardiovascular disease.

If you have modified your diet from testing your tolerance to foods, tuned up your exercise, you're sleeping well, and feel like you're handling stress well, you may benefit from IF. I recommend having all of those pieces in place before you look to IF. Then begin in phases.

Start with "fasting" between meals and an overnight "fast" of at least 12 hours. Close the kitchen after dinner. I'm often asked, "What's a good after dinner snack?" Crickets. There isn't one. This isn't about going to bed hungry. It's about looking back on your last meals and making sure you've had enough. You really shouldn't be hungry 2-3 hours after dinner if you had fat, protein, fiber and some quality carbohydrates at your meal. Going between meals and overnight without food is important to your gut and hormone balance.

If you're a grazer going from meal to snack without a break, stop. You may never be really allowing hormones and digestion to operate optimally. Eating more small meals throughout the day to boost metabolism is a myth. In fact it backfires and encourages fat storage. Your body will never need to dip into stores if you're constantly feeding it.

Next, increase your overnight fast by an hour or two.

Increase your fast so that your eating window is 8 hours. You don't necessarily reduce your intake, but listen to your body. Hunger and satiety signals will help you know what your body needs. Ironically, when you fast, most women report that they will experience less hunger and more alertness.

Beware of reliance on coffee during your fast. If that's how you get yourself through a morning fast you're elevating your cortisol and missing the point. You can have a couple cups then shift to water.

Beware of going overboard. It's all too easy to get caught in wanting to accelerate weight loss and skip the return to eating more. If you constantly eat less and less, your body will burn less. If enjoying meals with friends and family are a part of long-term health for you as it is for most people, fasting full time is going to feel pretty limiting. If you can't do it for life, I would always question whether starting it is a good idea.

Long-term negative effects of IF are still unknown. For midlife women more susceptible to the negative effects of stress, IF is definitely taking stress imposed by dieting to a new level. So many initial IF studies are done on mice, and young adults, primarily males, showing IF can match results of other restrictive dieting and in some cases exceed those results.

We've known for years dieting works, short term, until it doesn't. The metabolism slowdown that occurs often results in regains bigger than losses. Don't go on a diet. Adapt a diet you can do for a lifetime.

Last, what about exercise during a fast? Logic might tell you that your body will be forced to burn fat if you're not eating. That's true. The problem is both muscle loss and comfort. You need to exercise to keep muscle during a fast.

It's harder to use fat for fuel. Your intensity and any potential pleasure from exercise may suffer. You won't be able to work as hard (and therefore you'll expend less energy during and after) and your "feels like" scale of how hard you're working is going to go up. If you've not bonded with exercise, this can kill your motivation.

94. Be a Picky Eater

Consumer reports found unacceptable levels of heavy metals in randomly tested popular protein powders. This is a problem considering protein shakes are often consumed multiple times daily. You know the program: have a shake for breakfast, a shake for lunch, and a healthy dinner. Labels in some states are required to carry warnings and yet even then not all producers are compliant. Even food and safety agency representatives don't agree what is and is not acceptable. So it's up to you.

Protein shakes are not your only exposure to toxins, but toxic protein powders are avoidable. You are exposed to heavy metals through foods to some degree, too. If you consume foods highest in heavy metals frequently you increase your toxic exposure. For example, sunflower seeds and spinach, as well as shellfish, potatoes and rice can be high in cadmium in part due to cadmium-containing fertilizers.

Decrease toxins and decrease your weight loss resistance. Those toxins get stored in fat making fat more stubborn to lose. Important internal organs like your liver and kidney get overtaxed with heavy metal consumption. You are a finely tuned machine that wants to hum along with all cylinders firing. If anything slows down your metabolism, looking good and feeling great becomes much more challenging.

Review your diet and rotate foods frequently. Shop organic whenever possible. Rotate spinach with kale, microgreens, and other salad greens regularly. Flip your rice for quinoa.

This is perfect example of "healthy" not always being healthy. Repeatedly eating the same thing again and again can rob you of micronutrients that come from eating a variety of foods and it can increase toxic exposure.

Check ingredients on labels carefully. Ask about testing of the products. Responsible producers are aware and will confirm third party heavy metal testing.

I use Flipping 50 plant-based shakes, beef-based shakes, and whey and in rotation. I have a breakfast shake daily. A second shake might fit in on a rare occasion, say we're shooting episodes of Flipping 50 and I'm making one on set or we're too tight on time to break. I try not to have too many days like that. I know that buying for one fear of having food spoil before you eat it but I make a habit of buying three different types of greens instead of the monster size spinach only. I eat spinach every other or every third day and plan meals and snacks so I'm not defaulting to some of my favorites: shrimp, sunflower seeds, sun butter, and spinach too frequently.

I included a link to the Food and Drug Administration's list of food sources of heavy metals in the resources section.

94. Down Dog Blues Away

Even if you don't have the mojo to get breathless or lift weights – yet – you may find a nice mood boost on your mat. Twice weekly yoga sessions can help. A study of primarily female subjects average age 43 showed just eight weeks of Hatha decreased signs of depression during the study. Researchers were focused on the yoga-depression relationship but found subjects also enjoyed a healthy boost in their self-esteem and self-efficacy too.

That self-efficacy may be just the shot you need to move you to the next step in goal setting and goal getting. It may be the non-judgmental nature of yoga helps your tendency to constantly compare and measure performance. It's likely a combination of components in yoga from the accepting environment, to releasing physical tension, to the distraction from other stressors or rumination -that overthinking about things women often do that provide positive mood benefits.

Hatha yoga is a fairly gentle flowing yoga, easily modifiable for a wide variety of needs. You can find a studio, DVDs, or streaming options for yoga you can do right in the convenience of your own home.

The advantage of a scheduled class however is that you've made a promise by registering not just to the instructor but also to yourself. Make the dates with a specific times and days to show up. If you opt for home exercise, make sure you choose an accountability partner or coach to help you keep that promise to yourself.

Surround yourself with others doing what you're doing or what you want to do.

96. Lose With Yoga

There's no need to turn the heat up to 110 for hot yoga or to jump from pose to pose in a power yoga session for a yoga practice to help your weight loss. If you're struggling to make other exercises a regular routine, or to change dietary habits, yoga might be the answer. Yoga is not notorious for high calorie burning or the "after burn" that lingers and boosts metabolism for hours that other fitness activities boast. Still, you may want to reconsider if you've skipped over it.

Yoga does have a positive weight loss effect on both overweight and normal weight participants. For subjects who had both tried other means of weight loss and failed and normal weight participants not set out to lose weight, yoga resulted in weight loss. Their comments were reviewed by researchers who wanted to determine why.

Mostly female subjects with an average age in the mid-fifties reported that their weight loss was a result of shifting to healthier eating. They described their experience using terms like "becoming more mindful" and "conscious about what and why" they were eating. It wasn't intentional but occurred as they progressed in their yoga practice.

Food cravings decreased in many of the yoga participants. Admitted emotional eaters in the study reported that they felt less need to fill themselves with food because they had less emotional void. Stress reduction, other study participants said, helped them make healthier choices.

The sense of community in yoga classes was also an influence for participants. They reflected about becoming the people they spend time with and wanting to emulate their instructor and classmates with the same healthier attitude and choices.

Are you surrounding yourself with a community going the direction you want to go? Learn more about support with Flipping 50's Café membership.

http://bit.ly/2y7BLGZ

97. Age Stronger

If you've flipped into your 60s (or 70's and beyond), your fight for the right to keep muscle is real.

However, it's been said that muscle loss is a natural part of aging. I call B.S.

Muscle loss is a natural part of less exercise and/or ineffective exercise. Let's don't lie to ourselves. When I'm not as happy with my exercise results as I was 10 years ago, I can point to not being as active on a daily basis as I was 10 years ago. (Make no mistake. I'm not saying just do more. You need to change the way you exercise and do LESS but more purposeful exercise on a consistent basis, not just turn up the random acts of fitness.)

You can maintain your muscle, and in fact, you can gain muscle at any age. You do need to apply some specifics to your routine. You can't just simply "exercise" and expect results. Any more than you could throw flour, sugar, cocoa and eggs together in random order and expect to get a cake. (That, by the way is not a suggestion.)

Just like medicine has a dose-response relationship, so too does exercise. Or let's use wine. One glass, Debra is funny. Two glasses, Debra thinks she's funny and laughs at her own jokes. Three glasses, nothing tonight or tomorrow is funny.

When researchers examined the dose–response relationship of exercise they found some very specific things to be true about strength. Please know that when we're talking about strength, we're also talking about increased lean muscle, better body composition, and better metabolism.

The variables that provide the greatest and most rapid results in strength are these:

- 60 seconds between sets
- about six seconds per repetition
- twice a week training frequency
- two to three sets per exercise
- seven to nine repetitions per set
- 4 seconds between repetitions

There are some big take-aways here. Rest more between both sets and between repetitions. Four seconds rest is going to feel like a lifetime if you're used to lifting and lowering and lifting until you're finished with a set.

Another big take away is twice a week is more beneficial than three times a week. Researchers were very specific about this. While there was little difference between two or three sets during each workout, the clear winner was twice a week as opposed to one and the often recommended three times a week. It is important you understand that less frequent higher quality exercise can lead to more optimal results. Recovery can't be ignored. The seven to nine repetitions are "to fatigue." It isn't a suggestion to simply stop when you get to nine. You want to be earning that rest and recovery.

Try this one! Try the 6 seconds for each repetition so it's 1-2 seconds to lift and 4-5 to lower. Rest 4 seconds between repetitions.

Use the recording in your book bonuses to guide you through it.

98. Avoid "I've Tried Everything" Syndrome

This is the #1 most common frustration I hear from midlife women. You're willing to change, you're taking advice, and you're trying it but it's not working.

You wind up going back to your default habits. What always worked before was calorie counting. What always worked before was just doing more exercise. What always worked before was ________________ (fill in the blank). With fluctuating hormones, changes in metabolism and body composition, however, what used to work probably won't again.

Random efforts at random changes tend to get at best random results.

If you want to consistently get repeatable results you have to operate like a scientist. Collect data. There's two parts to scientific knowledge. A scientist first investigates. They observe what's going on now. That, for instance, is where I start clients with a three-day food and activity log. I ask them not to change anything but to record everything.

By looking over patterns of activity and associating energy levels and weight or performance we can determine how current habits are positively or negatively work for you. Whether its digestion, or weight, or belly fat, that are getting in the way of your best life, we focus on what we can change and test.

Then we determine which specific variables to test. If you're going to learn how certain diet changes affect you, you need to keep others the same. If you want to know how various workouts influence the results you want, you'll want to change one thing at a time. You start with a reset. Get a clean slate and it's easier to isolate changes.

Mary was diagnosed with osteoporosis. When Mary began her exercise program focused on avoiding more bone density losses we made one change at a time. This allowed forward progress without risk of injury. We start with one set of 8-10 exercises with a fairly high number of repetitions (20) twice a week. If we assess that's going well we increase to two sets after two weeks. Two weeks later if it's going well we increase the weight so Mary is only able to complete 15 repetitions.

Mary's program continues to progress until we have her to the number of sets (3) and the weight she can only do up to 10 times by alternating increases of repetitions or weight. We don't change both. We don't change frequency. If Mary has a negative response we'll know precisely what caused it and we can use that data to make our next step.

You never fail. It's all data. Nowhere else in our lives do we expect perfection from a single effort with a major overhaul. Scientists and inventors and entrepreneurs all fail and get up again more than they succeed. Without those fails there would never be predictable repeatable change for the rest of us to enjoy.

So determine what needs to be tested or changed. First.

In Mary's case it was exercise. In your case it may be nutrition. It could be sleep habits. Choose the target you want to improve. Then build an experiment around it. Track it. Measure progress. There's no failure with a scientific experiment. It's all data. You test it, collect information, and move to the next step.

I realize I've just given you dozens of what might feel like random things to do in the pages of this book. Take them one at a time and try them on. You're still in the dressing room, tags on. You don't have to buy any of them yet. Or do buy them. Take them home and leave the tags on. See how they work with the other things you have in your closet. You don't throw it all out and get all new; you add new pieces here and there.

If you want support organizing steps to make changes right now, and you are an action taker ready to rock her second half, make an appointment to talk about your options private or group options.

Schedule here:

http://www.scheduleyou.in/ZzFwszm

99. Facts Are Not Enough

Irrational passions might guide you more. Once you form an opinion it may be hard to change it. If you decided before you picked up this book, for instance, that diet changes don't work, or they don't work for you, even with evidence on the pages here showing otherwise, history says you may not change your mind.

Humans tend to have confirmation bias. We seek information that verifies what we already believe.

So, if you're thirsty for information that says you don't have to settle for the example of aging that you've seen in past generation, or you're unwilling to accept that weight gain is just a fact of life as you age... you may be loving the 98 flips that have come before this one.

If on the other hand, if you picked this up with strong skepticism you will find holes in much of the reason on these pages. You'll resist the idea that something so simple could actually change the way you age, your energy, or your weight. In fact, if you're over 50 you have been conditioned to disbelieve most of the things included in this book and the very idea that you can love your body and set new goals well into your 60's, 70's and beyond.

It's no wonder if you've fallen under the spell of accepting statements that end in "for your age," or you ask what percent body fat is acceptable at age 50 or 60 or later. (It doesn't change from the time you're 20, beautiful.) The norms and averages have changed, but what is healthy is the same. Why shoot for average? If average is your goal, this is not likely your book.

You can put this confirmation bias under faulty thinking. We all have our own irrational passions, ideas we grab ahold of and can't let go of. According to Stanford research begun back in the 70s confirmation bias is one of the most common types of faulty thinking. (Apparently we have many options to go down that path).

Your thoughts are not reality. But you may go to considerable lengths to try to prove they are.

Confirmation bias leads you to dismiss evidence of new threats to your current beliefs. I've taught both young and older adults in classrooms, lectures, and online presentations for 30 years. I've witnessed that anyone can be presented with a significant amount of research evidence, facts in other words, and respond, I don't believe that.

What they mean is "I don't agree with that," or "I'm not going to accept nor apply it to my own life." Facts are facts. I'm not telling a fictional story, it's research that happened and results that occurred.

Strong feelings about fitness or nutrition or how you can age don't happen based on knowledge as much as they happen based on other minds. Have you noticed the emerging trend, as of this writing at least, to join groups in Facebook? We join the groups supporting the habits and beliefs we already have or we want. We can actually get more smug and determined based on our thoughts being supported and backed up by a group. Even if those thoughts are wrong.

There's actually a rush of dopamine, a neurotransmitter that makes us feel good, when we process information that supports what we already believe. Oh, do we like to be right.

Reaching for a community of like-minded believers works for women. We like to collaborate more than compete. Don't take offense to that. We can certainly compete but we can also support while we do it. We lift each other up even in competition though.

We don't have an attitude of if one of us wins the rest of us lose. We realize that there is more room at the top of the podium. That, in fact, gets stronger with age. We aren't threatened by someone taller, thinner, who's graying more beautifully than we think we are. We're more hopeful about our own possibilities because of her.

Join our community. Give, get, and hang around other women flipping their second 50.

Hot, not bothered, we're going to rock this world.

References

1. https://www.ncbi.nlm.nih.gov/pmc/articles/PMC4217002/
   https://www.ncbi.nlm.nih.gov/pubmed/22402738
2. https://www.ncbi.nlm.nih.gov/pmc/articles/PMC1785201/
   http://www.huffingtonpost.com.au/2016/08/22/the-truth-about-lemon-water-on-digestion-and-detoxification_a_21456136/
3. https://www.ncbi.nlm.nih.gov/pmc/articles/PMC3569688/
4. https://www.ncbi.nlm.nih.gov/pmc/articles/PMC2290997/
5. https://www.ncbi.nlm.nih.gov/pubmed/28675917
6. https://nutritionreview.org/2013/04/medium-chain-triglycerides-mcts/
7. https://www.hsph.harvard.edu/nutritionsource/healthy-drinks/soft-drinks-and-disease/
8. http://www.backfitpro.com/documents/Spine-flexion-myths-truths-and-issues.pdf
   https://www.ncbi.nlm.nih.gov/pubmed/9854759
9. https://www.ncbi.nlm.nih.gov/pubmed/28409690
   http://journals.lww.com/psychosomaticmedicine/Abstract/2017/01000/Perceived_Stress_After_Acute_Myocardial.7.aspx
   https://www.ncbi.nlm.nih.gov/pubmed/28460563
   https://www.ncbi.nlm.nih.gov/pmc/articles/PMC3671133/
10. https://www.ncbi.nlm.nih.gov/pmc/articles/PMC3718776/
    http://www.mdpi.com/2072-6643/9/4/352/htm

11. https://www.ncbi.nlm.nih.gov/pmc/articles/PMC3201893/
https://www.ncbi.nlm.nih.gov/pmc/articles/PMC4394186/
https://www.ncbi.nlm.nih.gov/pmc/articles/PMC4633096/

12. https://www.ncbi.nlm.nih.gov/pmc/articles/PMC4924200/
https://www.ncbi.nlm.nih.gov/pmc/articles/PMC4208946/

13. https://www.caltonnutrition.com/micronutrient-master-class-how-to-compare-2-multivitamins-using-the-abcs-of-supplementation-guidelines/

14. http://ajcn.nutrition.org/content/early/2013/01/30/ajcn.112.050997

15. http://jn.physiology.org/content/109/5/1444

16. https://www.ncbi.nlm.nih.gov/pubmed/28205155
http://www.ewg.org/skindeep/top-tips-for-safer-products/#.WY7-Z62ZMcg
https://www.ncbi.nlm.nih.gov/pubmed/12608524
https://www.ncbi.nlm.nih.gov/pmc/articles/PMC3569688/
https://www.ncbi.nlm.nih.gov/pubmed/28975368

17. Dr. John Ratey, Spark: The Revolutionary New Science of Exercise and the Brain (2008)
https://www.ncbi.nlm.nih.gov/pmc/articles/PMC2249754/

18. http://jn.nutrition.org/content/130/2/272S.full
http://europepmc.org/abstract/med/2228407

19. https://www.ncbi.nlm.nih.gov/pubmed/25168533

20. http://news.mit.edu/2004/carbs

21. https://www.ncbi.nlm.nih.gov/pubmed/15212756
https://www.ncbi.nlm.nih.gov/pubmed/23179202

22. https://www.ncbi.nlm.nih.gov/pubmed/26894275
https://www.ncbi.nlm.nih.gov/pubmed/19001042?dopt=Abstract

23. https://www.ncbi.nlm.nih.gov/pubmed/12975635

24. https://www.ncbi.nlm.nih.gov/pubmed/15111494

25. https://www.ncbi.nlm.nih.gov/pmc/articles/PMC2908954/
https://foodbabe.com/2012/02/19/be-unconventional-stop-drinking-with-your-meals/
https://www.ncbi.nlm.nih.gov/pmc/articles/PMC2908954/

26. https://www.ncbi.nlm.nih.gov/pubmed/24901744
https://www.ncbi.nlm.nih.gov/pubmed/27695975
https://www.ncbi.nlm.nih.gov/pmc/articles/PMC4063875/

27. https://www.ncbi.nlm.nih.gov/pubmed/28303052

28. https://cellsciencesystems.com/education/research/inflammatory-symptoms-immune-system-and-food-intolerance-one-cause-many-symptoms/
https://www.ncbi.nlm.nih.gov/pubmed/28740352
https://www.ncbi.nlm.nih.gov/pubmed/19087366

29. https://www.ncbi.nlm.nih.gov/pubmed/28724171
https://www.ncbi.nlm.nih.gov/pubmed/25274610
https://www.ncbi.nlm.nih.gov/pubmed/28771949
https://www.ncbi.nlm.nih.gov/pubmed/28758133

30. http://psychology.oxfordre.com/view/10.1093/acrefore/9780190236557.001.0001/acrefore-9780190236557-e-157
https://dash.harvard.edu/bitstream/handle/1/3196007/langer_excersiseplaceboeffect.pdf?sequence=1

31. Back Mechanic: The Step-by-step McGill Method to Fix Back Pain Stuart McGill (www.backfitpro.com) Sept 2015

32. https://www.ncbi.nlm.nih.gov/pmc/articles/PMC3703169/

33. https://www.ncbi.nlm.nih.gov/pmc/articles/PMC1476070/
https://www.ncbi.nlm.nih.gov/pubmed/28847480

34. https://www.ncbi.nlm.nih.gov/pubmed/9760324
https://www.ncbi.nlm.nih.gov/pubmed/28804437

35. https://www.ncbi.nlm.nih.gov/d/?term=A+Role+-

for+Sweet+Taste%3A+Calorie+Predictive+Relations+in+Energy+-Regulation

36. https://www.ncbi.nlm.nih.gov/pubmed/22948807
https://www.ncbi.nlm.nih.gov/pubmed/28117717 (peanuts allergy)

37. https://www.spine-health.com/blog/how-hyperextending-your-knees-affects-your-spine

38. McGill, S.M. (2007) Low back disorders: Evidence based prevention and rehabilitation, Second Edition, Human Kinetics Publishers, Champaign, IL, U.S.A.

39. https://www.ncbi.nlm.nih.gov/pmc/articles/PMC4530716/

40. https://www.ncbi.nlm.nih.gov/pubmed/28771085

41. https://www.ncbi.nlm.nih.gov/pmc/articles/PMC4517022/
http://jn.nutrition.org/content/139/2/264.short

42. http://wurtmanlab.mit.edu/static/pdf/993.pdf

43. https://www.ncbi.nlm.nih.gov/pubmed/24549028
https://www.ncbi.nlm.nih.gov/pmc/articles/PMC4776937/
https://www.epa.gov/choose-fish-and-shellfish-wisely/fish-and-shellfish-advisories-and-safe-eating-guidelines
https://www.fda.gov/Food/FoodborneIllnessContaminants/Metals/ucm393070.htm
https://www.ncbi.nlm.nih.gov/pmc/articles/PMC4427717/

44. https://www.ncbi.nlm.nih.gov/pmc/articles/PMC3354005/

45. https://www.flippingfifty.com/if-eating-paleo-beat-ms-should-you-consider-it-too/

46. https://www.ncbi.nlm.nih.gov/pubmed/24718534
http://www.brainlife.org/fulltext/2001/kelly_gs010600.pdf

https://www.ncbi.nlm.nih.gov/pmc/articles/PMC3545242/

47. https://www.ncbi.nlm.nih.gov/pubmed/16843606

48. https://www.ncbi.nlm.nih.gov/pubmed/28676855

49. https://bmcpublichealth.biomedcentral.com/articles/10.1186/1471-2458-14-726

50. https://www.ncbi.nlm.nih.gov/pubmed/26676059
https://insights.ovid.com/pubmed?pmid=27300110

51. http://journals.plos.org/plosone/article?id=10.1371/journal.pone.0062593

52. http://www.backfitpro.com/pdf/selecting_back_exercises.pdf

53. http://jap.physiology.org/content/early/2011/04/25/japplphysiol.00210.2011

54. https://www.ncbi.nlm.nih.gov/pubmed/25748168
https://www.ncbi.nlm.nih.gov/pubmed/28819746

55. https://www.ncbi.nlm.nih.gov/pmc/articles/PMC2968119/

56. https://www.ncbi.nlm.nih.gov/pubmed/28460563

57. https://www.ncbi.nlm.nih.gov/pubmed/21849912
https://www.ncbi.nlm.nih.gov/pubmed/20555276

58. http://www.nejm.org/doi/full/10.1056/NEJMoa0707302#t=article

59. http://www.bmj.com/content/357/bmj.j1745
https://www.ncbi.nlm.nih.gov/pubmed/26551910

60. http://www.backfitpro.com/pdf/selecting_back_exercises.pdf

61. http://www.nejm.org/doi/full/10.1056/NEJMp1504023#t=article
http://stm.sciencemag.org/content/6/218/218ra5
http://journals.plos.org/plosone/article?id=10.1371/journal.pone.0015591

62. https://www.ncbi.nlm.nih.gov/pmc/articles/PMC1361002/

63. https://www.ncbi.nlm.nih.gov/pubmed/21159787

64. http://ajcn.nutrition.org/content/early/2013/01/30/ajcn.112.050997
http://www.cmaj.ca/content/189/28/E929
https://www.ncbi.nlm.nih.gov/pmc/articles/PMC2892765/

65. https://www.ncbi.nlm.nih.gov/pubmed/11782267

66. https://www.ncbi.nlm.nih.gov/pmc/articles/PMC3578432/

67. https://www.ncbi.nlm.nih.gov/pubmed/28702808
https://www.ncbi.nlm.nih.gov/pubmed/20703499

68. https://www.ncbi.nlm.nih.gov/pmc/articles/PMC3894304/

69. https://www.ncbi.nlm.nih.gov/pubmed/22306437
https://www.ers.usda.gov/data-products/adoption-of-genetically-engineered-crops-in-the-us.aspx

70. http://jap.physiology.org/content/early/2016/05/09/japplphysiol.00154.2016

71. https://www.ncbi.nlm.nih.gov/pmc/articles/PMC3048776/

72. http://www.ncbi/nlm.nih.gov/pubmed/12537959 http://www.ncbi.nlm.nih/2299589

73. https://www.consumerreports.org/cro/2012/04/protein-drinks/index.htm https://drlindseyberkson.com

74. https://www.ncbi.nlm.nih.gov/pmc/articles/PMC5052677/
https://www.ncbi.nlm.nih.gov/pubmed/?term=Declines+in+Sexual+Frequency+among+American+Adults%2C+1989%E2%80%932014
https://drlindseyberkson.com/oxytocin-new-hormonal-kid-clinical-block/

75. https://www.ncbi.nlm.nih.gov/pmc/articles/PMC4983298/

76. https://www.ncbi.nlm.nih.gov/pubmed/25223963
http://www.nature.com/npp/journal/vaop/ncurrent/full/npp2017148a.html?foxtrotcallback=true

77. https://www.ncbi.nlm.nih.gov/pmc/articles/PMC3354005/

78. https://www.ncbi.nlm.nih.gov/pubmed/24766579

79. http://journals.plos.org/plosone/article?id=10.1371/journal.pone.0062593

80. https://www.ncbi.nlm.nih.gov/pmc/articles/PMC3183816/

81. https://www.ncbi.nlm.nih.gov/pubmed/15972618

82. https://www.ncbi.nlm.nih.gov/pubmed/28542024

83. https://www.ncbi.nlm.nih.gov/pmc/articles/PMC3880087/

84. https://www.ncbi.nlm.nih.gov/pubmed/23792939

85. https://www.ncbi.nlm.nih.gov/pubmed/28539176

86. https://www.ncbi.nlm.nih.gov/pubmed/28736622

87. https://www.ncbi.nlm.nih.gov/pubmed/21492428
https://www.ncbi.nlm.nih.gov/pubmed/26885697

88. https://www.ncbi.nlm.nih.gov/pubmed/28786812
http://www.rmmj.org.il/userimages/704/0/PublishFiles/704Article.pdf

89. https://www.ncbi.nlm.nih.gov/pubmed/28886820

90. https://www.unm.edu/~lkravitz/Article%20folder/epocarticle.html

91. https://www.ncbi.nlm.nih.gov/pubmed/18091021

92. https://www.ncbi.nlm.nih.gov/pubmed/27339435

93. https://www.ncbi.nlm.nih.gov/pubmed/27810402
https://www.ncbi.nlm.nih.gov/pubmed/28106818
https://www.ncbi.nlm.nih.gov/pmc/articles/PMC4960941/

94. https://www.consumerreports.org/cro/2012/04/protein-drinks/index.htm
https://www.fda.gov/downloads/food...totaldietstudy/ucm184301.pdf

95. https://www.ncbi.nlm.nih.gov/pubmed/28301561
https://www.ncbi.nlm.nih.gov/pubmed/28917367

96. https://www.ncbi.nlm.nih.gov/pubmed/27594890

97. https://www.ncbi.nlm.nih.gov/pmc/articles/PMC4656698/

98. http://www.wikihow.com/Conduct-a-Science-Experiment

99. https://www.newyorker.com/magazine/2017/02/27/why-facts-dont-change-our-minds

Other Programs and Services
by Debra Atkinson

Flipping 50 TV

The Flipping 50 TV show is available right on the flippingfifty.com site. Just hop over and start watching as I answer real questions, from real women just like you.

I answer questions about what to eat, how to move, and how to fit it all into the rest of your busy life.

Plus, I share coupons and juicy specials with our Flipping 50 TV viewers from time to time!

We've shared cool fit fashions, exercise tools for home or travel, skin care, protein shakes, and more. It's all so that Flipping 50 viewers can feel good exercising, love the body they live in now, enjoy cooking and eating at home, and have amazing skin.

Here are just a few of previous seasons show titles:

- Why You're Exercising and Still Can't Lose Weight
- Prevent Back Pain (and Get A Flat Belly and Look Thinner)
- Get Motivated and Stay Motivated
- Exercise Less and Have the Body and Energy You Want
- Firm and Tone After Weight Loss
- Exercise for Stress Reduction
- Fatigue-Fighting Exercise Solutions

Flipping 50 podcast

Start listening now at https://www.flippingfifty.com/podcasts/ or you'll also find the show in iTunes. I'd love it if you'd leave a rating!

The once-weekly (with a few special editions) audio show features expert guests and me solo giving you juicy insider tips for education, motivation, and inspiration. I filter through all the confusion, conflicting, and overwhelming information and bring you what's relevant to YOU.

Popular recent episodes:

- Happier, Thinner, and More Energy Easier Than You Think
- Stop Sit Ups, Save Your Spine, Flatten Your Belly
- Bone Density, Osteoporosis, and Exercise After 50
- Finding and Keeping Your Motivation
- The Weight Training and Fat Loss After 50 Formula
- Flipping 50's The Art of Change: Habits This New Year
- Time for Habit Change with Dave Smith

If anything catches your eye, just enter the title in a search and it will come right up.

https://www.flippingfifty.com/podcasts/

Flipping 50 blog

Twice a week I post a written letter to my Flipping 50 fans. Sometimes it's like a diary entry sharing my training for an event and how I balance hormones by changing the traditional training program to fit right now.

Sometimes it's a heated response to something I see online that is perpetuating myths that take you further from your goal.

Sometimes I'm inserting video and explaining clear how-to for exercises along with the all-important (to me, and I hope to you) why they're important to you.

The categories I cover vary. The topic is always the same. You, you, you.

- Exercise
- Hormones
- Nutrition
- Mindset
- Sleep
- Stress
- Rest & Recovery

Stop by if you prefer to read.

https://www.flippingfifty.com/blog/

If you'd rather listen while you commute or workout, the Flipping 50 podcast is a perfect option.

Flipping 50's 28 Day Kickstart and The After 50 Fitness Formula for Women courses

How to choose between:

28 Day Kickstart

- 4 Live group coaching calls with Debra
- Content and Q and A every week
- Short, quick program with fast results (7-14 lbs. is average loss)
- Private Facebook community for sharing tips, challenges, questions between
- Bonuses for early adoption: video workouts, recipes, mind-set & program prep, and a private SOS call with Debra
- Your personal nutrition blueprint
- Lifestyle habits for women in peri-menopause or post menopause
- Optional upgrade: **Fast Flip coaching** (see below)

The After 50 Fitness Formula for Women

- · Do–It-Yourself (DIY) self-paced course
- · 12 months access to modules
- · Education-based program dives deeper into what to do and why

- Email support coaching you to stay on track through 8 modules
- Private Facebook group for community interaction
- Bonus Module 9: resources for exercise (not a workout component) and more
- New Bonus: Bone Health course (regularly $49) inside (Sept. 2017)
- Trial CAFÉ membership after course completion
- Optional Upgrade: Private **Fast Flip coaching** (see below)

Fast Flip coaching Upgrade (by invitation only)

- Available exclusively for current program students
- Program content serves as the foundation of calls and goals
- Custom weekly goals for 12 weeks/90 days
- Private brief weekly coaching with Debra
- a fraction of full VIP coaching (1/4 regular rate)

Flipping 50's Exercise Videos

You Still Got It, Girl

Muscles in Minutes

The Whole Flip

How to choose between:

THE WHOLE FLIP (DVD only) http://bit.ly/2ydhstw

- 4 DVDs professionally pressed products guaranteed to play
- A complete fitness program with cardio, strength, core, special joint care and even a special kitchen prep session
- For women who are able to move quickly, get up and down from the floor
- A lower impact cardio boxing still allowing higher intensity
- 10 and 20 minute "flips" to do solo or to add together
- Support with schedule planning, nutrition for success, getting started & progression, and tracking (delivered in email immediately with your order)
- New 2017

YOU STILL GOT IT GIRL (digital only) http://bit.ly/2zcXSf0

- 4 full length warm-up to cool-down strength workouts (45-60 minutes)
- strength-only workouts with core exercises

- · Delivered one per week for four weeks in email
- · No log in and no overwhelm of content day one!
- · Cheat sheet for each video for a workout with or without the video
- · Each workout based on specific goals: metabolism, bone density and fat loss, balance and performance, posture
- · Instruction rich
- · Downloadable to your computer then device

MUSCLES IN MINUTES (digital only) http://bit.ly/2yeEbF8

- 10 videos for quick, effective strength (only) workouts
- Super short segments (6-12 minutes) to combine or do solo
- Fit your time and your goals with body part specific videos
- Choose one, two, or three to fill your available time or goals
- Downloadable to your computer then device
- Two optional upgrades: cardio/mobility video set and a PDF book with exercise images, how to tips, modifications, and progression suggestions

Private VIP Coaching

This is the choice if you want lifelong change, big juicy goals, and you want VIP service along the way. You get full access to me for:

- Daily exercise planning right down the sets, repetitions, warm ups cool downs and core exercise.
- Daily nutrition coaching for realist goals that fit your home, travel, and hosting needs.
- Meal planning and recipe support whether you're flexitarian, vegetarian, or vegan.
- Weekly coaching calls for support, progression, and collaborating on next steps.
- Daily habit support to start or stop with flips that are doable, realistic, and proven.

Jump in for 90 days or the whole flipping 365 and save almost 50% off while you get more:

- Access to any programs
- Access to Café membership
- Reduced rate success kits (protein shakes, fiber, mint greens)
- Retreat time with Debra in Boulder Co for up to 3 days (train in the mountains, get one-on-one face time for strength training, yoga, running, biking, swimming, hiking, Pilates, etc.: we'll create a customer retreat for you)

About Debra Atkinson

Debra Atkinson has over three decades experience as a successful fitness entrepreneur, university lecturer in kinesiology, and international fitness presenter. She is a bestselling author and speaker with roots in Iowa and wings in Boulder, Colorado.

Her mission is twofold:

1. To raise the glass ceiling on expectations about aging and bust myths about menopause and midlife for women
2. To raise the quality of service in the fitness industry provide more and better options for you

She presents to leading fitness industry associations including IDEA, NSCA, Can-Fit-Pro, ICAA and Athletic Business and contributes to many of their periodicals. She is a frequent contributor for Huffington Post, ShareCare, Prime Women, LivingBetter50, and Easy Health Options and others. She's been consulted for articles in USA Today and Prevention Magazine regarding women's health through the exercise-hormone connection.

She is the creator of the web-based Flipping 50 TV show and Flipping 50 podcast and leads dynamic workshops live and online or with private clients that teach women how to love the body they live in and build confidence for every aspect of life with flipping fit foundation. This is her third book for the flipping 50 audience.

Flipping 50 was recently recognized as one of the top 15 blogs for over 50.

She can be reached at:
Https://www.flippingfifty.com

Or speaking site
http://www.debraatkinson.com

Facebook:
https://facebook.com/flipping50tv

Twitter:
https://twitter.com/flipping50tv

YouTube:
https://www.YouTube.com/allagesfitness

Instagram:
https://instagram.com/flipping50tv

If this book has been valuable for you would you leave a rating on Amazon? I would so appreciate it. If you find anything that needs correcting or that you want to comment on otherwise would you share that with me so I can fix it? support@flippingfifty.com

Made in the USA
Middletown, DE
08 December 2017